THIN
from
WITHIN

Jack D. Osman

Hart Publishing Company, Inc. ● *New York City*

COPYRIGHT © 1976 HART PUBLISHING COMPANY, INC.
NEW YORK, N.Y. 10012

ISBN. NO. 08055-1151-2
LIBRARY OF CONGRESS CATALOG CARD NO. 75-13431

MANUFACTURED IN THE UNITED STATES OF AMERICA

Contents

Preface

You may very well be asking yourself, "Why another weight control book?" Diet books are available that appeal to almost every appetite—books to help you lose weight quickly, others to take inches off your measurements, and still others that claim to tell the truth. Books have been written by psychiatrists, sportscasters, psychologists, scientists, nutritionists, popular writers, and medical doctors. Most of these weight control books are information oriented; that is, the author is interested primarily in "telling." Some are sensationalistic— the author is interested in "yelling" (often about how little he knows). And a few are interested in "selling"—the newest weight-control gimmick.

Thin from Within has been written with you, the dieter, in mind. In each chapter you will be asked to complete self-directed learning strategies. These learning strategies, which have been tested in actual weight-control classes, will give you clearer insight into your own values—an essential first step in weight loss, since it is a person's values that, ultimately, guide his behavior. This practical, "you-centered" approach is much like a workbook. The answers you write down will serve as a dietary diary, to be reread now and then as a source of continued motivation.

Thin from Within will also warn you about diet plans that are unworkable, poorly balanced, or downright unsafe. The information is documented so that you may pursue your own

4

areas of interest and determine the validity of what you are reading.

This book will help you lose weight by reducing the gap between what you know about dieting and what you do about it, between what you say about dieting and what you ultimately practice. Many people *know* a lot better than they *do*. The cigarette-smoking doctor knows he should not smoke, yet he continues to do so. Something in his makeup motivates him to continue the practice, even if it makes him feel guilty. As we all do sometimes, this doctor is displaying value confusion—he knows one thing but does another.

Many people are not determined in their own minds about what they value. Perhaps this is because we live in a society that expects us to accept without question the values of "authorities." However, if some belief is going to guide your life through time and space, that belief should be the result of your own free choice. If you are following a certain diet only because your doctor prescribed it, you will often find yourself cheating when you are not under the watchful eye of your spouse, or parents, or other authority influence. Unless you freely choose to follow that diet, you will never succeed.

Throughout this book I have taken the values clarification approach. The advantage of this approach is that it will help you formulate what you believe is right for your own life at a particular point in time, thus inclining you more toward consistency—to *do* what you feel good about and believe in, to follow through on what you say. Instead of continually announcing that one of these days you're going on a diet, you will begin now to modify your behavior, increasing the correspondence between what you think and what you say, what you say and what you *do*.

Some of the responses requested in the exercises may appear too simple or trite to record; others too difficult or personal. I encourage you to go ahead and write these answers down. Writing is a relatively permanent record, and you tend to think more critically about your answers before you begin to write. You may even find that this is the first time you have ever given thought to these questions. Occasionally you will be asked to go back and read over what you wrote at an earlier time. You may be surprised at what you wrote. Frequent reactions are: "Did I say that?" "Gee, I've sure come a long way since then!" "Hey, those ideas are pretty good." "I forgot all about that!"

This book does not pretend to be a panacea, or a form of therapy. *Thin from Within* is intended to be a mirror in which you can look at yourself and at your dietary habits and goals. In order that you may engage in critical thinking and positive action about weight control, I offer the following pages for your consideration and use. Good luck.

NOTE

Throughout this book the anonymous person has been referred to as he. This is not to imply that only males have a weight problem, or to slight females in any way. The decision was reluctantly made in the absence of any feasible means for resolving the indefinite pronoun matter. Care has been taken to avoid stereotyping, and it is hoped that the thrust of the book will be recognized to be essentially human and neither primarily male nor female.

Acknowledgments

The author wishes to express his sincere appreciation to all those who gave him encouragement and feedback during the four years this book has been in preparation—to friends, colleagues, and my best critics—the students—thank you.

To Carolyn Westbrook, Towson State College graphics department, a special thanks for her artistic touch.

Sincere gratitude is expressed to Judy Wederholt whose editorial know-how helped me say what I wanted to say.

To my family, I would like to express my thanks for their patience and understanding.

This manuscript has seen seven typists and proofreaders, and I would like to thank each of them: Ginny Colbert, Donna Holland, Susan Flack, Susan Moore, Isabel Stabler, Carol Mercogliano, and Sharon Morey.

To all of these people, and to all of you whom I will only meet in the pages of this book, I wish:

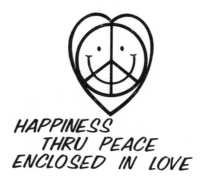

HAPPINESS
THRU PEACE
ENCLOSED IN LOVE

To Scott and Brooks

whose

love of movement

is my

movement of love

Thin from Within

If you are interested in winning at losing, have you ever considered getting thin from within? Many of today's dieters are only concerned with what they look like from the outside. They dream of how they will look when they have reached their goal weight. Little attention, if any, is given to what is going on inside their bodies, much less inside their heads. Getting thin from within demands that you use your whole being to help you reach your goal weight—your physical, mental, emotional, and spiritual resources. Getting thin from within relies on your willingness to take a hard look at what's going on in your head and your heart while you are following a weight-control program. For unless you get your head together, any weight loss you achieve will only be temporary.

Carl Rogers, therapist and author of many books on counseling, has stated: "All human behavior is exquisitely logical." Surely there are many valid reasons why people eat too much and exercise too little. You can change the external circumstances and even temporarily modify your behavior; however, unless the change is supported from within your head, even the most effective behavior modification program will not survive the test of time. You need to stop losing the game of weight control and start winning at life.

Becoming thin from within is a rational process of getting your head together. Lifelong weight control involves more than just balancing your diet. It requires a lifelong balance of self-direction. Thin from within means you will no longer make excuses for what you are, what you feel, or how you look. Once you have gotten your head together, the substantial weight loss that will follow may strike you as the least of your gains.

MOTIVATION: THE KEY TO WINNING AT LOSING

To lose weight permanently, you have got to be motivated. Your degree of motivation is directly correlated to the amount of weight you will lose and keep off. If your reasons are short-term—to fit into a swim suit for your vacation—chances are that you will only experience a short-term weight loss. Yo-yo dieting, with your weight fluctuating up and down, is hazardous to your health. You must be willing to commit yourself to a lifelong weight control program. Don't be alarmed by the sound of a "lifelong" program. Almost everyone practices some form of weight control throughout life. To maintain a desired weight instead of going up or down, you will simply be more aware of your program, at least initially. Even as you begin to work toward your desired weight, it is important to set up a nutritionally balanced diet *and* activity plan that you feel good about and can make a routine part of your life.

EXAMINE YOUR REASONS FOR WANTING TO LOSE WEIGHT

Rank in order of importance your reasons for wanting to lose weight. Try for at least three distinct reasons. Think your way through to the real reasons, not the fancy ones you give other people. State, describe or explain each one in a short sentence.

1. _____

2. _____

3. _____

4. _____

Look at what you have written down. Are these reasons strong enough to modify the eating habits you have followed for years? Will these reasons motivate you to appreciate and meet the need for body movement? Are you willing to walk regularly? Even to perspire? Regularly? Are you willing to minimize your use of such laborsaving devices as automobiles, elevators, escalators, golf carts, etc.?

How serious is your motivation to reach your desired weight? The battle of the bulge is a constant war. At the sure and steady rate of a one-to-two pound weight loss per week, you must be willing to spend months reaching your desired weight. Above all, you must have faith in the program and persist in it. Between 85% and 95% of dieters fail to keep their weight off for more than a two-year period. Such a high rate of failure might lead you to think, "What's the use? I'll just put the weight back on again." But it all depends on how carefully you gauge your motivation for wanting to lose weight.

I once worked on a construction project with a man I'll never forget. He held down two jobs. Most days he got only four or five hours sleep, and one day a week he didn't get any sleep at all. When given the opportunity to work overtime, I never knew him to turn it down. An hour before work began he would set up the equipment on the construction site and fill the ice water containers. One day I asked this father of seven school-age children, "Where do you get the energy to keep going? How do you keep up your motivation?"

"Well," he replied, "some folks *want* extra spending money, and some *need* that extra money. Me? I've *gotta* have it! There are no choices open to me."

If you want to lose weight for some short-term reason, you are probably insufficiently motivated, regardless of how well-intentioned and sincere you may be. Even if you *need* to lose weight because of external social pressures or health reasons, your enthusiasm for a lifelong weight control program may eventually wane. Those who have successfully controlled their weight over long periods of time are people motivated by the internal *gotta* principle. In which category do you belong?

Three motivations for weight reduction follow. Circle the one which best describes your motivation. Date this chart and sign your name to it.

```
┌─────────────────────────────────────────┐
│                                          │
│         1.  I  WANT  TO                  │
│                                          │
│                                          │
│         2.  I  NEED  TO                  │
│                                          │
│                                          │
│         3.  I  "GOTTA"                   │
│                                          │
│                                          │
│   _____    _____        │
│      date            signature           │
│                                          │
└─────────────────────────────────────────┘
```

When you really *gotta* permanently lose weight, you will definitely have more than "a slim chance in a fat world."[1]

DO YOU REALLY NEED
TO LOSE WEIGHT?

"Sure, of course I do. Why would I be reading this book if I didn't need to lose weight?" The popular singer, Carly Simon, has a song that goes, "I haven't got time for the pain, room for the pain, or need for the pain." When you realize that most dieters cannot maintain their weight loss over long periods of time, you may decide that the natural mechanism you are fighting is just too overwhelming. Much pain, anxiety, and frustration can be avoided by not being obsessed with a goal weight that may just be too unrealistic *for you.* If you are a moderately active individual who is between five and fifteen pounds over your ideal weight and you have stabilized at this weight for longer than six months, then perhaps your present weight is your biological ideal weight. Counteracting this biological mechanism may require enormous quantities of social and psychic energies. Have you the time, the need, or the room for such pain?

THIS HAS GOT TO GO!

As best you can, draw a picture of yourself at your present weight. Perhaps it would be easiest to start with a stick figure and then add layers of muscle and fat to your appendages. Be sure to provide both a front and a side view. *(See page 14.)*

Looking at your drawings, and setting aside your artistic abilities or lack of such, how do you feel about yourself?

Have you ever really been happy with your figure?

_____

What parts of your body do you like most?

_____

What parts do you like least?

_____

FRONT VIEW	SIDE VIEW

In the exercise below, list one positive physical characteristic for every negative one.

THIS HAS GOT TO GO	THAT CAN STAY

VALUES, WEIGHT CONTROL, AND YOU

Your values are the stars that guide your life. They light your pathway and give you direction. Taken collectively, your values form patterns that you can steer by, regardless of the situation you find yourself in. When decisions need to be made, the person with clearly defined values makes the most appropriate choice consistent with his cherished ideas. Even when faced with many conflicting alternatives, the "together" person weighs the long- and short-term consequences and then decides on a course of action. Talk is cheap—the valuing person is *action centered.*

When a dieter has chosen a weight control program, but is making little progress toward his desired weight, perhaps the difficulty is not in the program but in the *person.* Overweight people who are inconsistent, flighty, irresolute, and apathetic generally suffer from value confusion. They can't see the stars that could be guiding their lives.

> *Such persons seem not to have clear purposes, to know what they are for and against, to know where they are going and why. Persons with unclear values lack direction for their lives, lack criteria for choosing what to do with their time, their energy, their very being.*[2]

People who are confused about where they are headed will blindly follow almost any plan promising a solution. As the old saying goes, "If you don't know where you're going, any road will take you there." Unfortunately, most of the roads available seem to lead dieters around in circles or up and down the scale of yo-yo dieting.

For too long those concerned with weight control have

taken only a nutritional or medical viewpoint. The low success rate of these approaches suggests that something must be missing. In the past, doctors and nutritionists have treated just the *problem*—usually with pills and panaceas—and have ignored the *person*. They have rationalized that the diet is the problem—change the diet and you have a solution.

Recently, the "in" trend for the treatment of overweight has been behavior modification. Behavior modification principles, or BMPs, have been very successful in changing the dieter's behavior. BMPs are an important part of this book. But even behavior modification is not a totally satisfactory approach. Its main concern is with behavior *results*, not behavior *origins*.

The person cannot be separated from the problem. The dieter cannot be separated from the diet. Behavior modification techniques affect the diet problem, but not the dieter person. Becoming thin from within involves the *whole* person. It implies that your whole life may need to be reevaluated before you can ever hope to win at losing.

Loneliness, boredom, frustration, fear, resentment, confusion, rejection, disappointments—these are just a few of the underlying reasons why people eat more than they actually need. Sure, you can semi-starve yourself for short periods of time and even reach your goal weight, but unless the root of the problem is dealt with, the weight will eventually return. A good weight control program may help you get thin but still leave you frustrated, bored, lonely and confused. A confused person—going in all directions, never knowing which stars to follow—within a thin body is not the goal of *Thin from Within*. Your task (if you should choose to accept the assignment) is to get yourself together—to win at life—while you concurrently engage in an intelligent weight control program.

Let's take a moment to record some of the things that may be going through your head at this point. Write down your major concerns about life, other than your weight problem.

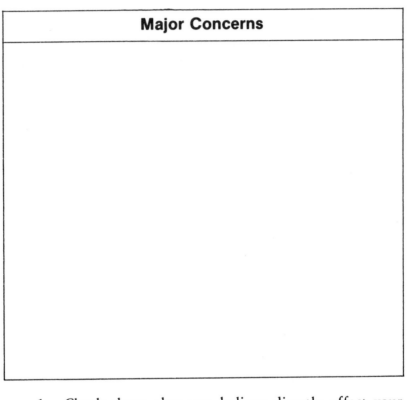

Major Concerns

1. Check those that you believe directly affect your weight control plan.

2. Star the one about which you'll try to do something constructive—*this* month.

3. List at least two things you might do about this problem.

   a. _____

   b. _____

4. Write down the name of one person who may be able to help you with this problem.

5. Write a letter to that person and explain what it is you would like help with. (It is often easier to communicate with someone about personal matters in a letter. Once the ice is broken, you will probably gain the confidence to deal with the person face-to-face.)

_____
                                                      date

Dear _____,

PRESSURE VALVES

When a goal, a need, or a drive is blocked, frustration generally results. Have you ever taken the time to identify how you deal with frustration, particularly when it's diet-related?

A pressure valve is a way to let off steam in certain situations. Below are listed some methods commonly used in dealing with frustration. If your methods are not listed, write them in the blank spaces.

Of all those listed, including those you have written yourself, rank order your five most frequently used pressure valves.

Pressure Valves

_____ I analyze the situation.

_____ I go on a snacking binge.

_____ I get depressed.

_____ I take some action to relieve the source of the frustration.

_____ I forget about it by doing some manual labor.

_____ I forget about it by going off somewhere alone.

_____ I cheer myself up by telling myself that the situation isn't really as bad as I think.

_____ I talk it over with someone.

_____ I express my frustration in my behavior, by acting very uptight or blowing up about something else.

_____ _____

_____ _____

_____ _____

Now code your five most frequently used pressure-valves according to the following criteria:

1. Write C next to those that you consider to be constructive.

2. Use a D to indicate a destructive pressure valve.

3. Write 0 next to a pressure valve that is cyclic in nature; that is, the pressure is temporarily relieved, but the problem will probably return.

4. Write X next to those pressure valves that you plan to avoid in the future.

5. Star those pressure valves that you will use in the future when faced with frustrating situations.

VALUES CLARIFICATION

Einstein characterized the age we live in as "a perfection of means and a confusion of goals." Modern life is complex and confusing. The communications media bombard the dieter with suggestions as to what is desirable, what is right, and what is worthy. Today's dieters are finding it increasingly bewildering, even overwhelming, to decide what is worth valuing and what is worth one's time and energy. At the same time, they want the kind of instant results to which our fast-moving world has accustomed us.

People who are unclear about what direction they would like to take in life often lack a system for filtering out the useless and the harmful. Without this filtration mechanism people find it difficult to make choices that are appropriate at any particular point in their lives. A filtration mechanism makes the decision-making process easier by providing a consistent, reliable reference point by which to orient oneself.

It is important that you have a clear idea of what you want for yourself when you decide to involve yourself in the weight control process. Consequently, much of *Thin from Within* is predicated on helping you see more clearly the stars that guide your life.

The values clarification process[3] has been charted in the following way:

CHOOSING: 1. Freely.

2. From alternatives.

3. After thoughtful reflection on the consequences of each alternative.

PRIZING: 4. Being happy, proud, pleased; cherishing the choice.

5. Being willing to publicly affirm the choice.

ACTING: 6. Doing something about the choice.

7. Repeatedly, as a pattern of life.

This seven-step process of valuing has been used in weight control programs. Consistently applied, it has helped people reduce the gap between what they say and what they do—and thus has helped reduce their weight as well.

CHOOSING, PRIZING, ACTING

Once you have chosen freely to embark on a weight control plan, you should then carefully consider which diet to choose.

In their book, *How the Doctors Diet,* Peter and Barbara Wyden have elaborated on more than twenty plans that physicians themselves practice.[4]

Obviously, then, there are many workable alternative plans from which to choose. Which plan will *you* select? What do you *prefer* in a weight control plan? What do you *know* about the plan that you choose to follow? Before you make your choice, investigate each plan's workability, nutritional adequacy, and safety.

For example, if you consult a bariatrician—a "fat" doctor who treats overweight primarily through prescribing pills (amphetamines, thyroid, diuretics, laxatives, digitalis, or barbiturates)—have you considered the possible long-range consequences of this alternative—its cost, as well as the psychological and physiological dependence on drugs that might result?

If a plan forbids you to eat your favorite foods, are you prepared to follow that diet as a lifelong program?

It is worth the time and effort it takes to decide intelligently on a program that will affect the rest of your life.

Meditate about your answer to each of the following questions:

Are you happy about the idea of beginning a diet?

Are you willing to make the necessary sacrifices?

Do you feel good about the weight control plan you have chosen?

Have you developed enough confidence in the plan to be glad you are following it?

When you feel good about going on a diet, you are likely to

affirm your decision when asked about it. You will, in all likelihood, be willing to make your position known to others.

If you are ashamed of being on a diet, or if you do not affirm your choice when asked, you may have started on a plan that you do not value too highly.

If you value the need to diet and the diet program you choose, you will *act* upon the plan, not just *talk* about it. In fact, the plan will direct your eating patterns and your entire life will be affected by the plan you select. If you feel good about your diet plan, you should find it less difficult to practice it as a pattern of life. The most successful weight control plans do not restructure eating and activity habits precipitately. Over time, new habits are gradually built up which can be adopted not just for the time being, but as a pattern of life.

Intelligently *choosing* a weight control program, *prizing* it and, because there are good reasons for prizing it, *acting* on it—this is getting *thin from within*, the values clarification approach to weight control.

REFERENCES

1. Stuart, Richard and Davis, Barbara, *Slim Chance in a Fat World*, Carbondale: University of Illinois Press, 1972.
2. Raths, Louis, Harmin, Merrill and Simon, Sid, *Values and Teaching*, Columbus: Charles Merrill Publishing Co., 1966, p. 12.
3. *Ibid.*, p. 30.
4. Wyden, Peter and Barbara, *How the Doctors Diet*, New York: Trident Press, 1968.

Before You Begin

Hollywood and Madison Avenue have saturated our senses with the ideal of the young, slim, beautiful person. This conditioning has so strongly influenced the American mind that many of us automatically reject a partner whose figure is less than ideal.

The male, especially, foolishly believes that only a person with an attractive figure is likely to have an attractive personality. Rarely will he seek out a relationship with an overweight woman, even if she is an intellectual heavyweight, a sensuous lover and capable of the deep emotional intimacy for which he is searching. Unless the male consciousness is suddenly raised, the overweight woman's only chance with such a man is to reduce.

Conversely, many a woman is so repelled by a pot-bellied male that she is immunized to whatever charms may be concealed within those layers of fat. In our society, thin is in.

No wonder so many people are obsessed with their weight. Who wants to be rejected on such a superficial basis? The sad truth is that many overweight people come to accept the evaluation made by others and feel that their weight problem cancels out the good qualities of their minds and personalities. They dislike themselves, and see themselves as outsiders in a thin society. Is it necessary to suffer such agony? Can the fat person maintain his sense of security about his self-worth, or does his embarrassment about his physical appearance prevent him from relating to others?

Learning and thinking strategies or exercises are interwoven throughout this book. These strategies have one or more of the following four purposes:

1. To present you with information, opinions, situations, controversial points of view.

2. To provoke you to think through the relevance of the facts and opinions to *you*, at *this* point in your life.

3. To encourage you to express, *in writing,* your reactions. Since writing provides a relatively permanent record, you may more carefully think through what you really think and feel.

4. To give you the opportunity to reflect back over former responses, to see if and how they differ from your present responses. You should routinely date each strategy after you complete your answer.

Roaming Eyes

Imagine yourself in the situation presented below. Then answer the questions.

You're dieting, but are still more than fifty pounds above goal weight. You've just begun to believe that you can be appealing to the opposite sex despite your plumpness.

You're at a party, and you've engaged in several conversations. Although the conversations have been neither long nor intellectually stimulating, you're gratified that at least people don't seem to avoid you as they used to. But you notice that in all the conversations people just seem to be going through the motions. They talk trivia and rarely maintain eye contact. Their eyes roam continuously around the room.

Now you are talking to someone. Suddenly he spots an attractive, slender woman coming in the door. You feel you're getting the brush-off. He excuses himself, ostensibly to get a snack, but actually he makes a bee-line to meet the attractive person who just came in.

1. What went through your head as you read this passage? What did you feel?

2. Has this ever happened to you? How did you react?

3. Did you leave the party early? Say more.

4. Alone, back home, what did you do? How did your reaction express itself in your behavior?

5. If this situation were a common occurrence in your life, what consequences might such experiences have on your psyche?

6.   List several alternative courses of action that are open to you.

A Thin Value Structure for a Fat Society

Read the following presentation. Then answer the questions.

It seems somewhat inconsistent that society stresses the virtues of thinness and yet saturates our senses with advertisements for high-calorie foods. Many advertised edibles are not essential foods; they're more often empty calorie junk foods. If ad men are subtly encouraging us to consume their high-calorie goodies, then it would seem that we should be permitted to store those extra calories without being disapproved of by society.

In a society in which nearly 50% of the population has a weight problem, who is setting the standards? We can't win! If we succumb to advertising ploys, we submit to excess consumption of calories. When we gain weight, we are made to feel ugly and guilty because society values thinness. No wonder overweight people are frustrated!

1.   Have you confronted the inconsistency described here?

2.   What have you done in response to it?

3. Who *is* society, anyway? Have you felt yourself pressured by society? In what way?

4. Have you ever resisted society's pressure? Write about it.

THE CYCLE OF REJECTION

Because society has conditioned us to see thinness as desirable, overweight persons often feel like social outcasts. Clothes are designed for the slender build. Colleges have been known to discriminate against obese students in their admissions policies. Employment discrimination is also common.

Over time, the overweight person's feelings of rejection accumulate and lead to feelings of worthlessness, particularly if nothing is contributing to a sense of self-esteem. When profound enough, these feelings develop into unconscious feelings of self-hatred. Most people's psyches cannot tolerate self-hate, and they protect their psychological well-being by devising defense mechanisms. Some kind of escape hatch is needed to cope with self-hate.

The trouble is, escape hatches do not solve the problem; instead, they lead to further feelings of rejection as people react to the escape hatch behavior. For example, if the escape hatch is alcohol, the self-hating fat person may drink to excess whenever he feels depressed about the futility of his life. Another popular escape is food. If the overweight person turns to the kitchen for solace, as he has been conditioned to do, his negative feelings of rejection, worthlessness, and self-hate will be compounded by feelings of guilt over the failure to stick to his diet.

Alcohol, overeating, drugs, sexual promiscuity, avoidance

of intimacy—whatever the particular escape hatch, the pattern is the same: people react negatively to the escape behavior, the person's sense of rejection is reinforced, and so the cycle continues.

Cycle of Rejection

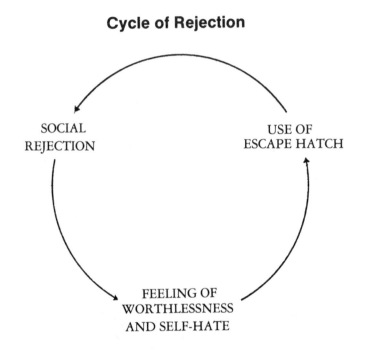

SOCIAL
REJECTION

USE OF
ESCAPE HATCH

FEELING OF
WORTHLESSNESS
AND SELF-HATE

OVERCOMING THE CYCLE OF REJECTION

The National Association to Aid Fat Americans (NAAFA) was formed by people interested in developing Fat Pride. At the monthly meetings, members try to help reduce each other's guilt and to improve their self-esteem.

When a person feels rejected, it is a totally encompassing feeling. This person feels bankrupt of any worth, self-esteem or self-love. Such emphasis has been placed on the overweight person's most apparent liability—his extra pounds—that he forgets the many assets and equities he has built up in other aspects of his life. Unfortunately, a healthy sense of proportion is hard to maintain in these circumstances. Sometimes the cycle of rejection becomes so intense that it begins to interfere with normal every-day functioning.

The exercise below is intended to remind you of the qualities you may have lost sight of in your concern over your physical characteristics.

On the left-hand side of the space below, list those qualities that you like about yourself. This is no time to be modest or vague. It's your time to brag and blow your own horn.

Down the right-hand side print the words *fat, overweight, obese, corpulent, paunchy, plump, heavy* or any other words that you feel are appropriate to your overweight condition.

This I Like	This I Don't Like

This exercise may strike you as silly, yet to complete it *in writing* is an important step in overcoming the cycle of rejection. Look at your list—you have many good and worthwhile characteristics. But because of society's obsession with thinness, they're all cancelled out in your mind by one supposedly overriding characteristic—excess adipose tissue.

"As you think, so you are." To break out of the cycle of rejection, focus on your positive attributes. It won't be long before you come to realize that, despite your weight problem (which you have the power to change), you have the same capacity for beauty and dignity as a thin person, the same ability to make worthwhile contributions to society, and the same right to enjoy yourself and your life.

As your feelings of self-worth increase, you will develop a more favorable vision of yourself—a type of self-love. Self-love is not necessarily narcissistic. You're not stuck on yourself if you love yourself. Many psychologists believe that self-love forms the basis for our capacity to love others. Without self-love, all other attempts at love will crumble for lack of a solid foundation.

Self-Love Continuum

If self-love could be plotted on a continuum, where along this line would you currently place yourself? Write your initials at the spot.

```
    :    :    :    :              :    :    :    :
 ───────────────────────        ───────────────────
SELF-LOVE           INDIFFERENCE            SELF-HATE
```

Think about three people you know who are thin or of normal weight, and about three overweight friends. Speculate as to where each of these people might be on the self-love continuum. What similarities or differences do you see between them and you that might be related to your various placements on this continum?

Print your name where you would like to be on this continuum and write the date by which you would like to achieve that end.

List several action-centered behaviors that you expect it will be necessary for you to engage in if you are to achieve your goal by the desired date.

1. _____

2. _____

3. _____

4. _____

SELF-LOVE AND SELF-KNOWLEDGE

One aspect of self-love is to recognize and accept your own feelings. Yet many of us, whether overweight or not, suppress our emotional responses to the behavior of other people, particularly if the response is hostile or resentful.

While struggling through a weight control program, we often come in contact with persons who generate strong feelings within us. Unexpressed resentment or hostility can produce within us a low-grade level of anxiety that can gradually erode our motivation and negatively affect more than just the weight control aspects of our lives. Direct confrontation with these feelings, rather than suppression of them as unworthy or invalid, is a more mature, self-loving alternative.

Resent-Demand-Appreciate[1]

In column one of the chart below, write the names of ten people with whom you regularly come in contact at home, work, school, or in your social life.

Name	Resentment	Demand	Appreciation
1.			
2.			
3.			
4.			
5.			
6.			
7.			
8.			
9.			
10.			

In column two, briefly state what, if anything, you resent about each person listed. For example, "I resent John because he is continually joking and teasing me about my weight."

Implicit in most feelings of resentment is a desire to have that person change his behavior. For example, "John, I resent your snide remarks and demand that you stop embarrassing me." Complete column three with the demand you would like to make of the people whose behavior you resent in some way.

If we walked in someone else's shoes for a few weeks, we might begin to understand why they behave as they do. In column four, write a statement that tells your appreciation for the other person's side of the story. For example, "I resent your remarks; I demand that you stop; but I appreciate your quick wit and your sense of humor—though not when it's at my expense."

"Resent-Demand-Appreciate" is a heavy strategy. Don't be frightened by what you write. What you feel is real. If you're involved in life, and have some self-love, the resentment you feel is normal. It can become a problem if it builds up to a point where it causes animosity, bitterness, and backbiting. Dealing with it openly is a much healthier alternative.

Are there any people on your list to whom you can show your chart? If you feel you can show it, do it gently, without hostility, and make sure to show them all the columns. The appreciation phase is important in reducing negative feelings on both sides.

LIFE ON A NO-RISK POLICY

Simon and Garfunkel, a popular singing duet, had a hit song entitled "I Am A Rock." The song told of a person who built defensive walls around himself for protection against a callous, hurtful world. He renounced friendship, love, and laughter.

Hiding out in an idealized world of books and poetry, he managed to cut off all contact with real people. He rationalized his behavior in the closing stanza of the song: "and the rock feels no pain and an island never cries."

Clearly the individual in the song has built up defenses against intimacy. Perhaps he has been rejected or hurt. As a temporary adjustment, withdrawal may be an understandable reaction to hurtful situations. However, if this attitude of isolation continues, the individual will miss out on a lot of good, reassuring experiences. Perhaps he really would like to reach out again, but is afraid of being rejected or hurt still another time. And so he continues to escape, to put up barriers against intimacy.

Have you ever met withdrawn people with painted-on personalities? They acknowledge your presence, yet remain cold, distant, and aloof. The walls they build around themselves trigger a negative reaction within us, which only confirms their belief in the necessity of defenses.

THE RISK-BENEFIT RATIO

Building walls as defenses against intimacy is analogous to the turtle's strategy of pulling his head back inside his hard shell for protection. But even the turtle has to stick his neck out eventually if he ever wants to get anywhere. To reap many of life's benefits, we too must stick our necks out.

We must be willing to take a chance. Initially, we may only risk a smile, a nod, or a friendly gesture to someone. As people react favorably to our nonverbal communication, perhaps we will begin to feel comfortable enough to speak up and make a casual observation or share some information.

Positive reinforcement for our verbal participation will lead to growing feelings of self-worth and confidence. Eventually, we may feel secure enough within ourselves to make other overtures, assuming leadership roles heretofore unimagined even in our wildest dreams.

THE PSYCHOTHERAPEUTIC VALUE OF PEOPLE

Sharing is an integral part of the opening-up process. Johari's Window, shown below, graphically depicts the potential benefits of human interaction through open communication.

The JoHari Window

	KNOWN TO OTHERS	UNKNOWN TO OTHERS
KNOWN TO SELF	Cell 1 OPEN	Cell 2 HIDDEN
UNKNOWN TO SELF	Cell 3 BLIND	Cell 4 UNKNOWN

Reprinted from *Group Processes: An Introduction to Group Dynamics* and *Of Human Interaction,* by Joseph Luft by permission of Mayfield Publishing Co., formerly National Press Books, 1970.

As you begin to share the hidden area of yourself with others, they too will feel comfortable sharing personal thoughts with you. Remember that this would not happen if both parties were unwilling to take the initial risk of being more open.

Feedback is an important and valuable part of this interaction. Feedback occurs when people feel comfortable enough to tell you things about your personality to which you yourself are blind. If you are willing to make the effort, gradual movement from the blind area to the open area will help you grow personally as you reduce poundage.

Taking the initiative to open up some of your hidden areas to others involves risk. The compensation for such risk taking is the added insight you gain into yourself as those with whom you have shared your hidden areas in turn reveal to you what they know about your blind areas. The depth of your sharing will be directly proportional to the magnitude of your growth. Without risk, there's not much chance of growth.

Thought Cards

On a regular basis (maybe daily, maybe weekly) write out a thought card. There are three basic rules for writing a thought card:

1. The subject must be something about which you feel strongly. It may be about any topic, of any length, in any style. It may even be a quotation that you particularly enjoy. The thought need not be restricted to your feelings about food or being overweight.

2. Date each thought you record.

3. Sign your name.

Collect these thoughts until you have accumulated about ten. Then go back over them and see if they reveal your attitude concerning life in general, or, more specifically, about weight control.

Ask yourself the following questions:

Upon rereading, which thought would you drastically rewrite?

Can you spot a pattern in the ideas that you stand for?

Are you genuinely proud of most of your thoughts?

Have you ever taken action related to the subjects of your most strongly-felt thought cards?

If you are ready to take a moderate risk, choose the thought card you are most proud of and share it with a friend.

CYCLE OF ACCEPTANCE

As feelings of self-worth develop, they slowly establish a stable base for self-love. Feeling more secure, the overweight person experiences a much less drastic need to escape, especially through overeating. As he begins to lose weight, he gets praised by family and friends, enjoying positive reinforcement from a formerly negative society. Warmed by these genuine gestures of acceptance, he is strengthened in his feelings of self-love. And so the acceptance cycle goes on.

Cycle of Acceptance

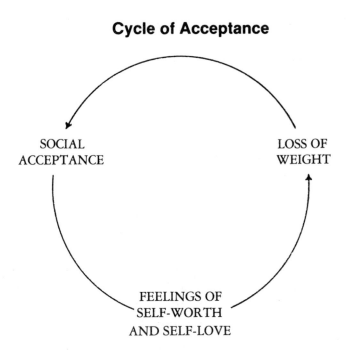

SOCIAL
ACCEPTANCE

LOSS OF
WEIGHT

FEELINGS OF
SELF-WORTH
AND SELF-LOVE

FROM SELF-ANALYSIS TO SELF-DIRECTED DIETING

How you feel about yourself will play a great role in how you feel about weight control. The key to winning at losing is getting yourself together—getting thin from within. Once you are paying attention to your own thoughts and feelings, sharing your successes, and doing your best to cope with defeats and bad times without slipping back into the cycle of rejection, your efforts at weight control will be only one part of a well-integrated process of dealing with your particular life situation. And because your weight control program is involving you as a whole person, your chances of success—at life and at weight loss—are much greater.

TWO CAUTIONS BEFORE YOU BEGIN

Before you undertake the program recommended in this book, there are two things you should consider.

First Caution: At this point in your life, is it safe for you to undertake a diet and activity program?

Be sure to have a physical examination before beginning any weight control program. Ask your doctor if you should be aware of any special restrictions in food intake or limitations in activity. People with special problems like colitis, ileitis, kidney trouble, or heart trouble may be advised not to attempt a weight loss program.

On the other hand, some persons who think they should be on a restricted activity program may, in fact, be encouraged by knowledgeable physicians to participate in a mild program of activity. Only your doctor can advise you in this area. His instructions should supersede those of any weight control plan you may read about.

I, ———————————— have checked with my doc-
         name

tor, ————————————, on ————————————; he has
       name   *date*

given me his approval to begin a diet and activity program,

being cognizant of the following limitations:

————————————   ————————————————
    date   *signature*

The Physician: Consultant or Cornerstone?

The following quotation is from the Foreword to the

Consumers Union Edition of Jean Mayer's *Overweight*. Read it and then answer the questions that follow.

> . . . *In considering a program of weight control, Mayer insists that the physician remain the cornerstone of therapy for the obese individual. Consumers Union agrees with Mayer in principle. The management of obesity is and will remain a medical problem. Decisions about a weight control program—who, when, how much—should be made by a physician, and the program executed under his guidance or with his knowledge. But, as Mayer himself states, many health professionals, including physicians, are poorly trained in nutrition and in the management of obesity. And, we must emphasize, physicians willing to treat obesity can range from the conscientious and well-informed doctor to the doctor who simply hands out a diet sheet—and even to the doctor who specialize in lucrative but questionable and sometimes dangerous procedures.*[2]

1. Do you agree with Jean Mayer that a doctor should be the cornerstone of a weight control program?

2. Do you agree with Consumers Union that many doctors are not adequately trained to handle obesity problems?

3. Would you ever consult a bariatrician—a doctor who

specializes in the treatment of fat patients? Say more.

4. How would you know whether the doctor you consulted about your weight problem was sufficiently qualified?

5. How adequate is your own knowledge about weight control?

6. List at least three sources of reliable weight control information.

Second Caution: Are you aware of the consequences if you fail to reach your desired weight?

Are you willing to take that risk? How determined are you to work to improve your eating and activity patterns? If you have been overweight for a long period of time; if you were overweight as a child; or if your occupation does not provide opportunities for you to be active, be prepared for a difficult struggle. Failure in a weight control program can set into motion the vicious cycle of rejection—rejection of self, rejection by society and friends, possibly even rejection of life.

Seriously examine your motivation before beginning a weight control program. Failure to follow the diet produces feelings of guilt, one of the most powerful elements in the cycle of rejection.

If you are not really serious about losing weight, perhaps

you had better wait until you *are* serious, rather than run the physical risk of yo-yo dieting and the psychological risk of getting stuck in the cycle of rejection.

REFERENCES

1. Simon, Howe, and Kirschenbaum, *Values Clarification,* New York: Hart Publishing Company, 1972, pp. 358-362.

2. Foreword to the Consumers Union Edition, 1969 (Editors of Consumer Reports) p. vi of Jean Mayer's *Overweight.* (Englewood Cliffs, N. J. Prentice-Hall, © 1968)

How Serious Are You About Losing Weight?

If you are interested in losing weight *permanently*, medical histories suggest that you only have a "slim chance in a fat world." Many diet plans can help you lose weight, sometimes even quickly. However, much of the weight quickly lost is water, not fat, so the loss is only temporary.

A worse pitfall is that deprivation dieting can, and often does, backfire. As the dieter approaches his ideal weight, he tends to slacken off and revert to his old eating patterns—often with enthusiasm, because for so long he has had to deprive himself of his favorite foods. When eating patterns are restricted more severely than the human constitution will tolerate, either the dieter will defy the restriction and eat as much as he wants of the forbidden food; or his continued frustration will result in neurotic patterns of behavior—sneaking food, deceiving himself, acting irritable.

To lose weight permanently, you need to modify the conditioned habits that caused your overweight. This means a sensible, long-term weight control plan. Nutritional reeducation is what the dieter needs, and this is where most popular diets fail. On a crash calorie-reduction diet, the dieter is generally instructed (somewhat dogmatically) to deprive himself of certain foods. These taboo foods are often some of his favorites, and may even fulfill certain social or psychological needs. It is no wonder that these are the very foods craved by the cautious calorie counter once he has won the physiological battle of the bulge. Before deciding that you can muster the willpower for a very restrictive diet, consider the following possibility.

ON-AGAIN, OFF-AGAIN DIETING

The average American goes on 1.25 diets per year, often going on and off with the changing seasons.[1] For some dieters, this up-and-down elevator approach could mean that the dieter's health is getting the shaft.

Yo-Yo Dieting

People who lose weight generally gain back much of the shed poundage during the same year. This on-again, off-again system of dieting not only results in frustration, but also in possible damage to the heart and other organs. Several authorities suggest that mildly overweight persons should remain that way rather than run the risk of damaging their health by this yo-yo dieting pattern.

An extreme example is cited by Peter Wyden in his book, *The Overweight Society:*[2]

> *Medical literature routinely notes cases of dieters who have spent years losing and regaining hundreds of pounds in what Dr. Jean Mayer, a noted Harvard physiologist, has called "the rhythm method of girth control." And sometimes the obsession to alternate between extremes of caloric excess and self-deprivation has led to the most tragic results. (The best known example is proba-*

*bly Mario Lanza, the "American Caruso," who once
enjoyed twenty-three egg omelets for breakfast. He
died of a heart attack at thirty-eight after a lifetime
of binge eating and binge dieting during which he
dropped, on at least one occasion, 100 of his 270
pounds.*

1.   How many times have *you* lost weight only to regain
     much of it?

2.   How did you feel about yourself after you gained the
     weight back, particularly if you had a difficult time
     reducing?

3.   On food-avoidance, calorie-restriction plans, once
     dieters reach their ideal weight they have a desire to
     go back to their old eating patterns and to consume
     the foods they have deprived themselves of. What
     alternatives are open to you in an attempt to avoid
     this yo-yo effect?

Diet After Diet

On the chart below, list the various diet plans or weight
control methods that you have tried.

Indicate the number of pounds you lost on each diet.

Score each plan according to the following code:

a.   Write "Dr." if the plan required medical
     supervision.

b.   Write "$" if the plan cost money.

c.   Write "T" for the plan that kept weight off for the longest period of time.

d.   Write "Rx" if the plan required that you use drugs.

e.   Mark the plan with an "X" if it proved harmful to your health.

f.   Draw a smiling face— —beside any plan you felt pleased with or happy about at the time you were following it.

Write down the best aspects of each plan.

METHOD	NO. OF LBS. LOST	CODING	BEST FEATURES

IF YOU'RE READY

If you are really serious about losing weight, let's make some realistic long-range calculations.

MY PRESENT WEIGHT: ————————

MY DESIRED WEIGHT: ————————

I NEED TO LOSE: ————————

Unless you are grossly overweight—seventy-five pounds or more—it is not recommended that you lose more than two pounds per week. There are several reasons for this. Generally, a weekly drop of more than two pounds reflects water loss, not fat loss. Since the body needs a certain amount of water to operate properly, it will either replace the lost water or operate inefficiently, leaving the dieter tired, weak, and lethargic. Besides, losing more than two pounds per week would require too drastic a reduction in your daily caloric intake and thus place too great a strain on your system and emotions. Finally, when calories are restricted too severely, chances are that your diet is poorly balanced.

Resign yourself to a long-term program. It has taken you months or possibly years of gradual gaining to reach your present weight. An almost equivalent amount of time should be taken to reverse the process. In estimating how long it will take to reach your desired weight, you must first determine by exactly how much you are willing and able to restrict your caloric intake over a long period of time.

To get a rough estimate of the number of calories that you are probably consuming to maintain your present overweight, multiply your present weight by the appropriate constant—16 for females, 17 for males.

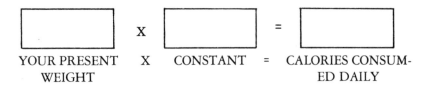

YOUR PRESENT   X   CONSTANT   =   CALORIES CONSUM-
    WEIGHT   ED DAILY

For contrast, also calculate what your caloric intake *will* be when you reach your goal weight.

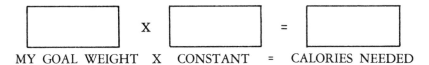

MY GOAL WEIGHT   X   CONSTANT   =   CALORIES NEEDED

The number of calories needed to maintain your current weight will change as you lose weight. Recalculate that figure every two weeks.

In order to lose weight at the rate of one to two pounds per week you have three choices:

1. Significantly reduce your caloric intake.

2. Increase your caloric expenditure through activity.

3. Mildly restrict your caloric intake *and* moderately increase your activity level.

I recommend a reduction in caloric intake of about 500 to 800 calories per day. *In addition* to the mild reduction in calorie intake, I recommend a mild increase in activity to help burn up an additional 200 to 400 calories per day.

If after about a month on this plan no results are seen,

then perhaps you are one of the five percent of the population blessed—or cursed—with a body system that is more efficient and economical than most people's. You require fewer calories to do the same amount of work as someone who is like you in all other respects. If this is the case, then it will be necessary to further restrict your caloric intake, and reduce the calorie-calculating constant to 14 or 15 for women; 15 or 16 for men. After a week or two at the modified level, you should begin to get observable results.

As you begin the program you may be overzealous and you may decide to restrict your daily caloric intake more severely than the suggested 800 calories. More drastic calorie restriction does not entitle you to forget about increasing your activity. *Mild activity is extremely important.* Ultimately the choice is yours, but whatever weight control program you eventually choose, you should be aware that a combined program of decreased calories and increased activity is the most successful over long periods of time. In the next few chapters you will be presented with information that will enable you to intelligently choose a diet and activity program that will take weight off safely, and keep it off permanently.

PLANNING AHEAD

To lose one pound per week you must cut your caloric intake, or increase your activity (preferably a combination of the two) by 500 calories per day. If you wish to lose 2 pounds per week, you need to show a deficit of 1000 calories per day. Reducing your daily caloric intake by *more* than 1000 calories per day is too limiting and too drastic a change for a long-term diet. To continue on such a restrictive program could discourage even the *gotta* motivated dieter.

Use the chart below to predict how long it will take you to reach your goal.

INCREASE ACTIVITY OR CUT YOUR DAILY INTAKE OF CALORIES BY	Days It Takes to Lose									
	1 lb	2 lb	3 lb	4 lb	5 lb	6 lb	7 lb	8 lb	9 lb	10 lb
100	35	70	105	140	175	210	245	280	315	350
200	17.5	35	52.5	70	87.5	105	122.5	140	157.5	175
300	12	24	36	48	60	72	84	96	108	120
400	9	18	27	36	45	54	63	72	81	90
500	7	14	21	28	35	42	49	56	63	70
600	6	12	18	24	30	36	42	48	54	60
700	5	10	15	20	25	30	35	40	45	50
800	4.5	9	13.5	18	22.5	27	31.5	36	40.5	45
900	4	8	12	16	20	24	28	32	36	40
1000	3.5	7	10.5	14	17.5	21	24.5	28	32.5	35
1100	3.1	6.2	9.3	12.4	15.5	18.6	21.7	24.8	27.9	31
1200	3	6	9	12	15	18	21	24	27	30

Weight Plan
1. Number of calories to give up and/or burn up daily: _____ 2. Number of days to lose 1 pound at that rate (see chart): _____ 3. Total number of pounds to lose: _____ 4. Total number of days to reach "D" day (desired weight). Multiply item 2 by item 3: _____

The number of calories you are willing to give up each day determines how rapidly your body will give up fat. To lose one pound, you need to lose 3500 calòries. If you cut 100 calories each day from your daily intake, you will lose one pound in 35 days, which will result in a loss of between 9-12 pounds in one year! If you cut 1000 calories each day from your daily intake, you will lose weight at a rate ten times faster, that is, one pound every 3.5 days, or about 100 pounds in one year!

Choose a date when you *gotta* conscientiously *begin* your weight control plan. Write it down here: _____

Count ahead the total number of days that it will take to reach your goal weight. Record that date here: _____

If you're really committed to this goal, complete the following contract.

Contract

I,_____ , do hereby contract to begin a weight control plan of restricting my caloric intake and increasing my activity by _____calories daily, beginning on _____. I am fully aware that at this rate, I will reach my goal of desired weight pounds in approximately_____days. I further realize that when I reach my desired weight on or before _____ , I still must continue on a sensible eating and activity program for the rest of my life if I am to maintain my desired weight.

_____   _____
date   *signature*

Make a copy of this completed contract and place it in a spot where you will see it regularly—on the refrigerator door, perhaps, or on your mirror.

THE IMPORTANCE OF FRIENDS

Once you feel comfortable with this contract, it is important that you share its contents with a "significant other"—some relative or friend whom you care about, trust, and respect. Ask him to countersign your contract, thereby indicating his support of your undertaking.

If you choose not to share the contract with someone right now, plan to do so in the near future. It's important to publicly affirm your choice to others—to let people know that you wish to make changes in your life. Their support and encouragement are extremely important. If you are shy about bringing up the subject, perhaps your displayed copy will provoke questions from those who see it.

YOU NEED ALL THE HELP YOU CAN GET

Support from the people with whom you interact is essential to your success. You need continual encouragement, feedback, and reinforcement. But your family and friends, as well-intentioned as they may be, may not know how to help. They too need to be informed. They need to know what to do and say, as well as what *not* to do and say.

The following hints will help your friends and family give you the psychological support you need for the duration of your struggle:

Hints For Your Friends and Family[3]

THINGS TO DO

> ** Learn the facts about obesity. Authoritative material is available through the American Medical*

Association's Council on Foods and Nutrition, and from local health departments.

*Develop an intelligent attitude to match the facts you have learned about obesity.

*Test your attitude by asking yourself: "Is my approach to the obese person one of love, indifference, or rejection?"

*Discuss the situation with people who have been obese and are now successfully practicing weight control; this can be an illuminating experience.

*Don't make a fuss when your obese friend or relative starts dieting successfully; take it as a matter of course.

*Establish and maintain a healthy atmosphere in the home, with a place in the family circle for the obese member.

*Encourage new interests and participate whenever possible in recreational or occupational activities enjoyed by your obese relatives or friends.

*Be patient and live one day at a time—obesity generally takes a long time to develop, and doesn't disappear overnight. Accept setbacks and relapses with equanimity.

*Recognize the psychological consequences of dieting. The dieter's temporary bad temper will subside as the individual stabilizes at his new weight.

THINGS NOT TO DO

Don't preach, nag, or assume a holier-than-thou attitude. This will probably cause the dieter to escape more and more into overeating.

Never use emotional appeals such as, "If you loved me, you'd lose weight." This only tends to increase feelings of guilt, leading to a need to overeat.

Your obese relative or friend is not a moral weakling. Do not take over his responsibilities, leaving him with no sense of importance or value.

Don't shelter the obese person from situations where food is served; this does not help him handle the everyday temptations of our society. He will have to learn to control his food intake.

Never extract promises or place your obese friend in a position where he must be deceitful. Promises are readily given and readily broken, intensifying his guilt-feelings and loss of self-respect.

Be sure not to argue with or put pressure on the obese person when he is overeating—his response will usually be negative.

Don't cover up or make excuses for him.

Try not to feel like a martyr because of the responsibility placed on you. This attitude usually is sensed by the already remorseful obese person.

Avoid standing in judgment of the method of dieting selected by your obese friend.

If you have children, never use them as tools or turn them against the obese member of the family in an attempt to force him to cope with his problem of overweight.

After your friend or relative has read these suggestions, have him sign the following contract:

Having read the above hints, I _____

                              name of friend

do hereby agree to practice these Things To Do, and refrain from use of the Things Not To Do to the best of my ability.

_____   _____

   date   *signature*

The "I Urge" Letter

Another way to involve your "significant others" in your commitment is to enlist their encouragement and support by means of the kind of letter shown on the opposite page. You may want to send such a letter to several friends whom you regularly see. Most people like to get mail. If they receive a letter from you asking for their support in your program, they will be sure to comment about it the next time they see you. You'll then have the verbal opportunity to share more of the details with them.

I Urge Variations

Send a letter or telegram urging an overweight friend or relative to join you in your diet and activity plan.

Ask a number of relatives and friends to form a system—a group of people whom you can turn to by telephone when temptation or depression threatens to overwhelm you.

Dear _____ ,

    Today I've decided to undertake a common-sense program of diet and activity to reach my ideal weight by _____ . Obviously, I'll need all the
                      date
help I can get. That's why I'm writing to you. I urge you to help me.

    Will you support me in my long-term venture to control my weight? I'll need regular encouragement and reinforcement from you. If you come across reasonable ideas that may be helpful, feel free to share them with me. I won't be offended. Talk with me about the specifics of what I'm doing to increase my activity and decrease my caloric intake. Join me for walks. With your encouragement, support, and reminders, I know I'll be more likely to follow through on my desire to reach my ideal weight.

                              Sincerely,

_____
                   signature

List at least three people to whom you will send such a letter. When you have written to them, enter here the date each letter was mailed.

Names		*Date*
1. _____		_____
2. _____		_____
3. _____		_____

REFERENCES

1. Wyden, Peter, *The Overweight Society,* New York: William Morrow and Company, 1965, p.8

2. *Ibid.,* p. 5.

3. Miller, Dr. Claude H., *The Psychology of Dieting,* Eleventh Edition, Long Island City: Dannon Milk Products, Inc., 1968.

Getting Psyched for Starting

None of the numerous hints compiled in this chapter is earth-shattering. Practiced collectively, however, these suggestions could easily result in a two-pound weight loss per week. As you will see, most of the suggestions are just common sense. Many of them you can perform right now with only slight modification of your normal eating and activity patterns. Some of the hints will be taken up again later in the book and dealt with at greater length.

As you read down the lists, write your initials next to every hint that you can begin to practice *right now* without any great stress or hassle.

SUREFIRE HINTS TO DECREASE TOTAL CALORIC INTAKE

_____ Resign yourself to the fact that weight control is a lifelong struggle. If you let down your guard, fat will creep back.

____✓____ For the next few weeks involve yourself totally in thinking, reading, and writing about weight control. You must arm yourself with as much knowledge as possible to win the battle of the bulge.

_____ ✓   Watch your total calorie consumption—that means that food and drink both count. If you are trying to create a permanently slim you, it is important to remember that the effect of calories is cumulative.

_____ ✓   Become a calorie counter. Learn the calorie content of the foods you most often eat and drink.

_____   Eat at least three meals per day. Skipping a meal often leads a dieter to snack heavily or eat too much at the next meal. Be patient. It may take several weeks to get used to eating breakfast. But breaking-the-fast is very important in regulating the appetite.

_____   *Eat slowly!* Chew deliberately. If you find yourself eating too rapidly, put your fork down after each bite of food. It takes twenty minutes for the appetite center in your hypothalamus to get the message that you are ingesting food. Until it gets that message, your brain will continue to send out hunger signals that you will respond to. If you are eating quickly, you will probably eat much more food than you need before your brain sends out satiation signals. To get a head start on your hypothalamus, you may wish to eat a small low-calorie portion of your meal ten minutes before you actually sit down to the main course.

_____ ✓   Drink a glass of ice water five to ten minutes before beginning each meal. This will temporarily reduce your hunger and make it easier for you to eat slowly. Your dentist would not like to see you chewing the ice, but sucking it is okay, and it gives you the illusion of something solid in your mouth.

_____ Start your dinner with a salad, but choose a low-calorie dressing and use it sparingly. Regular calorie dressings may be used, but only in quantities of, at most, one half your normal serving. Below are the calorie contents for one table-spoon of popular salad dressings in regular and low calorie form.

Dressing	Regular	Low-Calorie
Thousand Island	70	25
Blue Cheese	71	11
French	57	13
Italian	77	11
Mayonnaise	110	19

_____ Reduce your salt intake. Learn to taste food first before you grab for the salt shaker. Excess salt in your diet retains fluids in your body. Reducing your salt intake will cause a moderate loss of unnecessary fluids that you have been carrying around.

___✓___ Eat smaller portions of high-calorie foods. Get in the habit of preparing smaller portions.

___✓___ Give yourself a psychological advantage by using smaller plates. This will fulfill your psychological need to see a full plate while reducing caloric intake. It really works. Try it!

———— ✓   Purposely leave small amounts of food on your plate, even if it's only a few string beans. The clean plate syndrome has been the downfall of many a well-intentioned dieter. When there is just a little bit of food left on the plate, it should become your new signal to stop eating.

————   Think and talk about your feelings when you leave food on your plate. The mind plays tricks on us. We begin to think up reasons for eating everything. Talking with empathetic friends about your feelings will often help keep things in proper perspective.

———— ✓   Substitute skim milk (90 calories) for whole milk (165 calories for eight ounces), or 1% butterfat content milk (115 calories), or 2% milk (137 calories). Keep a record of how many calories you saved; then calculate how much weight those saved calories would have caused you to gain in a year. (100 excess calories per day will cause a 12-pound weight gain per year).

———— ✓   Keep a written record of the calories you save by sheer discipline, as well as those you save by the substitution method. Keep a running total of the calories you save daily. It will bring a smile to your face to know that you are making yourself thinner every time you save calories.

———— ✓   Have someone take your photograph at different stages of your diet. You may want to wear the same outfit each time. Place these pictures sequentially in your Diet Dairy (page 74). This will give you an excellent Before-After image.

_____✓_____ Cut down on fats, especially animal fats. Fat is the most concentrated source of calories—two and a quarter times more concentrated than carbohydrates. Trim most visible fat from the meat before you cook it. Cut off or drain all the remaining fat before you serve it.

_____✓_____ Eat smaller portions of meat. Per serving, meat contains more calories than any other food group, and most Americans consume far more meat than they actually need. Limit yourself to two servings daily.

_____✓_____ You need not eliminate bread from your diet. But use bread that is thinly sliced—it will provide fewer calories per slice.

_____ Bread provides significant nutrition, but be careful what you spread on it! Jelly (50 calories per tablespoon), apple butter (32 calories), margarine (100 calories), and butter (100 calories) provide few nutrients. Peanut butter (81 calories) does contain significant nutrients.

_____✓_____ Be careful how you prepare potatoes. Minimize you consumption of fat-fried potatoes—hashbrowns, home fries, French fries, potato sticks, and potato chips. Cut down on your normal amount of butter or sour cream on baked potatoes.

_____✓_____ Increase the amount of vegetables in your diet, especially the low-calorie ones. Besides providing bulk, color, and essential vitamins, they usually require you to chew deliberately, thereby giving the food message time to reach your hypothalamus.

_____ Use artificial sweeteners whenever possible and palatable.

_____ Drink diet sodas, if you must drink soda.

____✓____ Rediscover your taste for that inexpensive, zero calorie, non-intoxicating drink—water.

_____ Drink thin. Watch that alcohol! Next to fats, alcohol is the most concentrated source of calories.

____✓____ Minimize your intake of all fried foods. Whatever you fry absorbs the fat, and at 255 calories per ounce of oil or grease—who needs it?

_____ When it comes to desserts, it's not always feasible to abstain. After all, why should you? Don't eat the full serving—nibble at it, leave some in the dish, or use smaller dishes. Do everything necessary to exercise control over eating. Desserts can provide an exercise in resisting temptation. Have a successful workout.

_____ Don't eat while watching T.V. We tend to eat unconsciously and lose track of our total caloric intake when we become mentally engrossed in something.

____✓____ Don't fool yourself when you cheat! These calories *do* count. Be aware of the tastes you snitch during food preparation.

_____ Watch those leftovers! Beware of the I'll-just-finish-this-up attitude. You may not want the leftover food to go to waste, but if you eat it, it will go to your waist. Have someone else clean up after meals. Dispose of scraps by putting them into the garbage can, or wrap leftovers up for immediate refrigeration.

Plan your snacks by saving something from one of your regular meals—a piece of fruit, crisp celery, a glass of skim milk.

Use common sense to select low-caloric between-meal snacks. Plan snacks in advance and buy the necessary ingredients during regular grocery shopping trips. Snacks bought on impulse are almost always high-calorie.

Eat your snacks in the same room where you eat all your meals. This will help you realize that calories in snacks count just as much as calories eaten at meals.

Don't hold lengthy telephone conversations in the kitchen. It's too easy to nibble.

A large stalk of celery (without salt, peanut butter, or cheese dip on it) is an excellent snack for the weight watcher (5 calories per stalk).

Most raw vegetables are good nutritionally and low in calories. They also slow you down by making you chew more. Careful, though, about snacking on fruit. Most fruits are moderately high in calories. If you prefer, instead of eating fruit at a regular meal, save it for a snack.

_____ ✓   Black coffee and tea also have zero calories. Since both contain caffeine they may serve to pick you up.

_____ ✓   When you crave a sweet, eat a sourball (15 calories) or a lifesaver (5 calories). But try not to keep this candy in your pockets, purse, or other convenient spot.

_____ ✓   Rearrange the refrigerator. Display in front the foods you are least likely to snack on.

_____ ✓   Chew gum (6 calories a stick) when you get the urge to eat something. Sugarless (4 calories) is best.

_____ ✓   Mentally rank order the foods on your plate by calorie content. Eat the foods with the lowest calorie-content first. Perhaps you won't be so quick to consume those last few bites of high-calorie foods at the end of each meal, knowing they contain the most concentrated amount of calories.

_____ ✓   Budget calories for special occasions and holidays. This is not cheating; you're just eating calories that were allotted to you before. It _is_ cheating, however, to eat more than you actually saved.

_____ ✓   Make a point to eat with friends or family. Eating alone is a common mistake of the concerned dieter. We tend to eat more balanced meals when we eat with others. Conversation also slows down the fast eater, thereby giving that delayed signal a chance to reach the brain.

————✓—— When possible, buy food in exactly the quantity you plan to eat. That extra ounce you get for practically nothing for buying the larger size will probably show up around your waist. Ultimately, you must decide if that risk is outweighed by the price differentiation.

————✓—— Break the habit of treating or rewarding yourself with food. Reward yourself by feeling good about the calories you have saved.

————✓—— Weigh yourself only once a week. Always do it at the same time, on the same scale, under the same conditions. Menstruation may temporarily alter the water balance. Do not, however, cheat on your diet and then blame the weight gain on your menstrual cycle—you're only cheating yourself if you do.

————✓—— Be aware of the cues that trigger your appetite. If seeing food is the cue that sets you off, then keep food out of sight as much as possible.

————✓—— Wrap and seal things tightly and elaborately. Tape shut the lids of jars and tins. This maneuver will cut down on odor cues. Also, you may decide it's too much bother to unwrap and rewrap the container for a little nibble.

DRAMATIC HINTS TO KEEP YOU INSPIRED

————✓—— Buy a terrific outfit in the size that will be yours when you reach your goal weight. Hang it somewhere to serve as a constant source of visual motivation.

_____ ✓   Make up signs bearing mottos like, "You can do it"; "One day at a time"; "Bathing suit here I come"; "A word to the wide should be sufficient"; "Win the No-Belly Prize"; "How many did you save today?" Post them througout the house (especially in the kitchen).

_____   Hang pictures of thin people around the house. However, on the refrigerator door, hang a picture of a grossly obese person.

_____   Place a polyethelene see-through container in the front of the refigerator. Keep it filled with raw vegetables. Print on the container in big letters: EAT THIN SNACK PACK.

_____ ✓   Tape a sign on a full length mirror—"You are what you eat," or "What you eat today, you'll wear tomorrow." Pause long enough to read the sign and look at your entire body in a relaxed state. Now suck in your stomach, hold your breath and look again. Practice proper posture.

Eat the following low-calorie items when you want to snack or shake the mid-day blahs.

_____   ice cubes (0 calories)—much better to suck on than hard candies.

_____   radish (1 calorie)

_____   pickle (dill: 15 calories; sweet: 30 calories)

_____ raw green pepper (10 calories)

_____ raw carrot (20 calories)

_____ broth or consomme (10–30 calories per cup)

_____ lettuce (14 calories per 3½ ounce serving)

_____ cucumber (7 calories ½ medium pared)

_____ sugar (15 calories per teaspoon)

_____ popcorn with oil and salt (1 cup 65 calories)

_____ bouillon cube (5 calories)

_____ extra large green olive (5 calories)

_____ medium tomato (35 calories)

_____ pretzels (20 calories per five small sticks)

Eat a few of your meals seated in front of a mirror. Observe yourself and note in your diary your impressions about the characteristics, speed, style, patterns of your eating habits. Seeing yourself as others see you while you're eating can bring valuable insights.

Also note in your diary your feelings while doing this exercise. What were your reactions? Did you tend to change your eating behavior? Did you eat faster? slower? more carefully?

HINTS TO INCREASE YOUR ENERGY OUTPUT

_____ Know that the risks of creeping obesity are real

and that your motivation to counteract your inactivity patterns must be high.

_____✓_____ Learn about the benefits of increased activity, especially in relation to a weight reduction program.

_____✓_____ Develop an appreciation for the active life. Explore the different movements of which your body is capable.

_____✓_____ Engage in activities that involve the large muscles of the body, particularly the legs.

_____✓_____ Participate in activities that you enjoy. You'll be more likely to do them again as a regular routine.

_____✓_____ Don't think of this increased activity as exercise. It may bring back unpleasant memories of physical education classes in which calisthenics were used as punishment.

_____✓_____ Movement is the key to activity. Begin to move more whenever and wherever possible.

_____✓_____ Stand rather than sit when appropriate—you'll use up nine extra calories per hour. In addition, when you're standing you are more likely to move.

_____ Minimize your use of laborsaving devices. As the world enters an energy crisis, remember that energy in abundance is stored within your tissues. This potential energy can best be released through movement.

_____✓_____ Walk up steps; skip the elevators and escalators.

Walking is great for burning up calories. You can do it alone or with others. You can walk to get someplace, or just to take in the beauty of nature. Rain or shine, you can walk fast, slow, with long strides, on your toes, Swedish style, or with a bounce step. No two walks need be the same.

Park your car several blocks from your destination and walk the rest of the way.

Walk to the local shopping center. Think about how nice it will be not to have to look for a parking spot when you get there. If you must drive, park in the farthest section of the lot.

Instead of having the daily paper delivered to your house, walk briskly to the nearest newspaper stand and pick it up.

Surprise friends by walking to their house.

Learn to *stride*. Striding short distances can rejuvenate your spirit while you burn calories, and increase your fitness level.

 Ask others to join you in your daily program of striding. Good company makes striding more pleasurable.

Take a brisk walk half an hour after dinner. Walking will keep your metabolic rate higher than would collapsing on the sofa in front of the T.V.

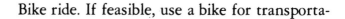 Bike ride. If feasible, use a bike for transporta-

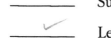

tion. People may stare at you, but haven't people already been giving you the stare that means, "Isn't it time you got back into things?" Besides, you're burning calories in place of gas. You're not polluting the atmosphere, and you'll be more likely to find a parking space.

_____ If you have a small lawn, use a hand lawn mower.

_____ If you golf, carry your clubs instead of pulling them on a cart. Stride after the ball between hits. The foursome behind you will appreciate your fast pace.

_____ If you enjoy calisthenics, do them to your favorite music, alternating between fast and slow music.

_____ Don't oversleep. Sleeping burns up fewer calories than any other activity. Within reasonable health limits, minimize the number of hours that you sleep. When you experience insomnia, get up and do some mild activity. The activity will tire you and increase your metabolic rate so that you will burn more calories when you do get to sleep.

_____ Beware of rainy days. Try to be active inside your house. Movement is the key. Remember, don't let bad-weather blues lead you to the refrigerator.

_____ Broaden your activity horizons. Watch your local newspaper for new activities to try. Call the local YMCA, YMHA, Physical Fitness Commissions,

Recreation Divisions, Sierra Clubs, Cycle Groups about activity schedules. Place your name on the mailing lists of service organizations so they can keep you posted on upcoming events. Get out of the house regularly. According to some scientists, even animals overeat because of boredom.

_____   When you go to the beach or pool, go to *swim*, not to sunbathe.

_____   When you see a vending machine, increase your walking speed until you are well past it.

Go back and star all those items that you would feel proud to do on a regular basis.

SUMMARY OF HINTS

If you are really serious about losing weight, you should have initialed approximately thirty-five of the surefire and dramatic hints. Activity not only burns calories but also helps to firm up sagging muscles. Therefore, you should have initialed at least fifteen of the hints to increase the amount and quality of your daily activity. If you choose a plan that does not involve a significant increase in activity, be aware of the consequences of your decision. In such a program, the only way you can lose weight (other than through surgery or drugs) is through strict calorie restriction. Your total caloric intake will have to be restricted severely (perhaps too severely) before you will make any significant progress. For example, if you choose to remain inactive and desire to lose two pounds per week through diet alone, you will need to eliminate 7000 calories from your normal weekly intake or 1,000 calories per day. If you were maintaining your present weight with, say, 2,000 calories, a 1,000-calorie reduction would be drastic, and might cause you to abandon the diet completely. It is difficult to have variety of foods and nutritional balance if your caloric intake is set at less than 1200 calories per day.

One-thousand-calorie diets often leave you hungry. Hunger causes pain. Pain has discouraged many a well-intentioned dieter. Therefore, if you choose not to increase your activity level, it may be necessary for you to adapt yourself to mild or severe hunger pains for the rest of your life.

If you are not willing to go hungry, some other sacrifice must be made. You must either increase your total activity level or remain at nearly your present weight. The choice is yours.

Diet Diary

Keep your own personal weight control diary. Write in it whenever you feel motivated, but aim for a daily entry, however brief.

Include diet plans, motivational quotes, calorie charts, pictures, anything you find relevant or helpful. Record the feelings—joys, pleasures, fantasies, frustrations, and failures—that you have experienced during your dieting. Save reliable articles and newspaper clippings. Look through this notebook on rainy days or when you get hungry. It will serve as a continual source of motivation.

*Motivational Quotes**

Here are some motivational quotes to get you started. Find—or make up—more on your own.

"No" Thyself!

What you eat in private
shows up in public!

Stick to your diet;
What have you got to lose?

The longer your waistline
The shorter your lifeline!

It's when you're on a diet
that the SECONDS count!

Are you "thick and tired" of it all?

The most attractive curves are the result
of three square meals a day!

A Minute on the lips;
A lifetime on the hips!

When you're a good chooser
You'll be a good loser.

Mirror, mirror on the wall,
Don't you ever lie at all?

The real winners
Are the big losers.

---

* Used with permission from the Diet Workshop's *The Busy Woman's Cookbook*, 1972

Whatever it is,
Don't eat about it.

Favorite Foods Profile

Using a reliable calorie-information sheet, keep a profile
of your favorite foods on the following chart. Add to it as you
think of other favorite foods and drinks.

Keep a record not only of what you eat, but where you eat
it, how you feel before eating it, with whom you are eating, etc.
All this information will help you identify firmly established
behavior patterns that must be recognized if you are to break
them. Continue this record for a week or more. You'll find the
more you write the less you eat.

Favorite Foods and Drinks	Portion Consumed	Calories	Where Consumed	Time of Day	Mood or State of Mind (bored, lonely, etc.)	What triggered the need for food? Whom were you with?

After completing the above chart, analyze the information as carefully as a scientist studies his data. Formulate three or more observations about yourself and your eating patterns.

1. _____

2. _____

3. _____

EATING AND EMOTIONS

Eating is more than just a physiological need. It involves our mental, social, spiritual, and especially our emotional dimensions. Food can provide security and contentment. Through eating we can express or conceal joy or frustration. Eating is a focal point of many social events and can unify a group of people. We devote hours daily to the purchase, preparation and consumption of food.

To lose weight, you must first be willing to achieve a psychological edge. You must train your mind and emotions to work *for* you, not against you. Becoming aware of your feelings about food and about eating is one of the first steps you must take. When you understand the roots of your behavior, you are well along the road to changing your inappropriate dietary habits.

Values Continuums

The following continuums are designed to help you find out about your own eating likes, dislikes, patterns, and habits. They are called values continuums because they indicate the wide range of values that is possible on any given issue.

The idea is to identify where you are in the here and now. Write your initials on the continuum at that spot. Then mark where you would like to be by writing your name at the spot that corresponds to your ideal position.

Note that the middle of the continuum scale has been purposely X'ed out. The middle of the road can often be an easy cop-out. It's like sitting on a fence made of whipped cream—sitting in the middle and avoiding movement in any direction makes you sink deeper into the cream.

A continuum identifies where you are at, and points out the distance from that point to where you would like to be. *You* are the only person who can initiate change.

Under each continuum, write a brief statement beginning with "I realize . . ." or "I will . . ."

Place

Where do you eat most of your meals?

EAT-OUT :   :   :   :   XXXX   :   :   :   : DINE-HOME
  EDNA   DINAH

Open comment:

Time

How much time do you spend preparing meals?

JIFFY   :   :   :   :   XXXX   :   :   :   :   ALL-DAY
JOAN   ANNA

Open comment:

Tastefulness

How much do you care about the taste?

THROW-
TOGETHER ——— :   :   :   :   XXXX   :   :   :   : GOURMET
THELMA   GRETA

Open comment:

Eating Cues

How do you know when to eat?

CLOCKWORK :   :   :   :   XXXX   :   :   :   : STARVATION-
CLYDE ———————————————— SIGNAL SID

Open comment:

Frequency

How often do you eat?

ALL-DAY :   :   :   :   XXXX   :   :   :   : THREE-MEAL
ALICE ———————————————— THELMA

Open comment:

Speed

How fast do you eat?

GULP-IT-DOWN : : : : XXXX : : : : CHEW-IT-SLOW
GORDON   CHESTER

Open comment:

Eating Habit

Do you eat whatever you're dished out?

CLEAN-PLATE : : : : XXXX : : : : LEAVE-LOTS
CLARA   LOTTE

Open comment:

Cholesterol

Do you avoid high saturated fat foods?

CHOLESTEROL- : : : : XXXX : : : : COULDN'T-
CONSCIOUS   CARE-LESS
CONNIE   CAROL

Open comment:

Eggs

Is this your dish?

EGG-SHUNNER :   :   :   :   **XXXX**   :   :   :   : EGG-LOVER
EDGAR   EGMONT

Open comment:

Sugar

How sweet do you like it?

POUR-DON'T- :   :   :   :   **XXXX**   :   :   :   : NEVER-TOUCH-
MEASURE   THE-STUFF
MARTY   STEPHEN

Open comment:

Dessert

Do you indulge?

DESSERT- :   :   :   :   **XXXX**   :   :   :   : DESSERT-
DESERTER   ADORER
DESMOND   DORA

Open comment:

Snacks

What do you fill up on between meals?

NUTRITION- :   :   :   :   XXXX   :   :   :   : EMPTY-
CONSCIOUS ——————————————————————— CALORIE
NED   ED

Open comment:

Walking

What do you use your legs for?

HIKING :   :   :   :   XXXX   :   :   :   : RATHER-RIDE
HYMIE ————————————————————————— ROGER

Open comment:

Physical Movement

How active are you?

SITTING :   :   :   :   XXXX   :   :   :   : ACTIVE
SAM ————————————————————————— ANDY

Open comment:

1. What did you learn about yourself from this exercise?

2. Are you happy with where you placed yourself on the continuums?

3. Would you reveal your position to friends? Even the positions of which you are not proud?

4. What can you do now to begin to move toward your ideal position on the continuums?

5. Go back and star the continuums that you want especially to work on during your weight control struggle. Record your ideas in your Diet Diary (*page 74*).

FEELINGS AND FOOD

Feelings are funny. They come and go like the wind. You rarely know where they come from or why they disappear. Yet, like the wind, feelings are indicators of things to come, particularly changes in your emotional climate. It is good to become sensitive to these passing weather fronts, for they often reveal patterns that, unless consciously dealt with, can work against success in losing weight.

Getting in touch with what you feel is not easy. Sensitivity to your own feelings takes patience, persistence, and practice. A few techniques might be helpful at the outset.

Here and Now Wheel

The Here and Now Wheel is designed to assist you in getting in touch with what you feel. Divide a circle into four portions, as follows:

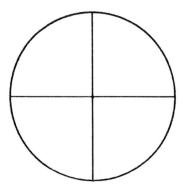

Within each of the four areas describe in one word a feeling that you are experiencing *here and now.*

When you are under emotional stress of a specific nature—like anger—one feeling seems to be overwhelming and it is often difficult to identify three other feelings you are experiencing at the same time.

It's interesting to discover that sometimes the feelings you write down appear to be in conflict with each other. That's normal. One reason for the Here and Now Wheel is to identify such diversity of feelings.

Select one of the four feelings you've written down and, in two sentences, describe, explain, or elaborate on that particular feeling:

_____

_____

_____

Writing captures those momentary, fleeting feelings and salvages them for future examination. Your two-sentence explanation helps to clarify one small but significant point in time.

After any joy, success, psychological up, do a Here and Now Wheel. Conversely, when you're down, bored, lonely, frustrated, angry, hungry, or just complacent, complete a Here and Now Wheel. Individually these wheels reveal little about you. But reviewed collectively they may reveal patterns that you should keep in touch with.

There are four good reasons for doing Here and Now Wheels regularly:

1. To help you get in touch with your feelings.

2. To clarify emotions that apparently conflict.

3. To encourage you to share your feelings with an empathetic listener, in the hopes of gaining more insight through feedback.

4. To give you the opportunity to think about feelings that normally are fleeting. After enough thought, you may eventually take the initiative and do something to express your feelings in action. We tend to think of negative feelings as unacceptable and we've been conditioned to bottle them up. This unnecessary repression of feelings can manifest itself in later life through ulcers, colitis, nerves, etc.

STAYING PSYCHED—WHAT TO EXPECT

There are a number of common pitfalls that the pound-shedding dieter will encounter. Knowing about them in advance should help you avoid these traps.

1. Think—don't just react—where food is involved. It is easy to fall back, unconsciously, to old eating patterns.

2. Don't become cocky. "I've been so good for the past month, a weekend eating spree won't hurt." Not so fast! Your splurge days should be very carefully planned. Many a well-intentioned dieter, ex-smoker, or ex-drinker has stood at the same crossroad. Cheating before you are psychologically ready could set into motion conditioned binge-eating responses that are almost irreversible.

3. Weddings, birthdays, and special holidays necessitate that your diet plan be flexible. Limit these special occasions to no more than once a month. If you maintain a calorie-restricted diet and increased-activity plan for 353 days, twelve days of prudent palate-pleasing should not upset your caloric homeostasis. On days following "planned cheating," engage in extra physical activity as a reminder of the price that must be paid to maintain energy equilibrium.

4. Watch out for boredom. Keep busy—in body and mind. An idle mind and body can be a dangerous combination in a society that conditions us to eat in response to boredom. If physical activity is inappropriate at the time that boredom strikes, telephone an empathetic friend and share your feelings. Or take out your Diet Diary (page 74) and try to put your feelings on paper.

5. Expect some depression. But don't give in to it. If depression is allowed to deepen, guilt may develop and the self-defeating cycle of rejection begin. Remember, when you're down emotionally it won't be long until you're back up again—provided you don't stop trying.

6. Adjustment to these new patterns of life will involve some risk—doing things about which you are unsure. Your feelings of hesitation or doubt are understandable, but unless you are willing to risk a little, not much progress can be made. Your success will come in direct proportion to the amount you are willing to risk.

7. Accept compliments as you begin to lose, but take them with a grain of saccharin. Compliments that go to your head often show up around the waist.

8. As your diet and activity plan progresses past the first few weeks of weight loss, you will hit a temporary period of remission or leveling off. Don't become discouraged. This is to be expected. Your body is making adjustments in its water balance. Although your scale will show no significant loss of poundage because of water retention, rest assured that calories of stored fat *are* being used for energy. Water will temporarily fill the empty spaces of the now-shrunken fat cell. Within a week or so, the body will readjust its water balance and will no longer need those pouches of water—provided your salt intake is within normal limits. (Most people use more salt than is considered healthy, especially those who regularly consume prepackaged, processed, or prepared foods.)

9. Sometimes on a calorie-restriction, activity-increase plan the scale will not reflect a weight loss, even though you *feel* and *look* lighter. Your own observations are correct, *and* your scale is accurate. You look and feel lighter in those once snug-fitting clothes because the increased activity has toned up your inactive and flabby muscles. As your muscles become stronger they will increase in density, weight, and sometimes in size. Your weight stabiliza-

tion is due, in part, to a much higher percentage of protein-water concentration in your lean muscle tissues than in your more buoyant excess fat tissue. Believe your feelings. You *are* losing fat. Things will balance out in a week or so and you will realize the reward for your efforts. Just remember, it's *fat* that makes you look and feel fat.

10. In your overzealousness, don't restrict your calories too severely. Consuming fewer than 1200 calories per day may cause your body to slow down its metabolism in an attempt to conserve its stores of energy. Your body doesn't know it's on a diet. It interprets the cutback in calorie consumption as a famine and deals with the situation by slowing down the rate at which it burns food. A good way to counteract your body's tendency to conserve energy is to increase your activity. Exercise speeds up your metabolic rate and thus balances the body's attempt to slow it down.

As you experience some of these pitfalls, jot down your thoughts and feelings in your diary. Note the situations and circumstances that you find most difficult. Keeping these feelings of frustration and discouragement locked up inside will eat away at your motivation. In writing down your feelings you are admitting that you have them, and preventing them from destroying you as a dieter.

The Proud Line

Your continued motivation will be sparked by the good feelings you have about yourself and your progress. The Proud

Line is a strategy designed to focus on the positive aspects of your weight-control behavior.

We are our own worst critics. We rarely take time to reflect on and feel good about our successes for fear of becoming self-centered. But healthy acceptance of accomplishments is an essential part of your weight control program.

Every day, write down one or more things you *did* for your diet and activity plan about which you are proud. Only *actions* count, not intentions. In this way you are reinforcing and rewarding *behavior.*

You may be proud that you took a walk or used the stairs rather than the elevator. Perhaps you feel good about resisting the temptation to raid the refrigerator for a snack.

Begin now. Record something that you did today that you can be proud of.

TODAY I . . . _____

_____

_____

Occasionally you will experience "down days"—days when you not only have no accomplishments to feel good about, but also do things you regret. It is worthwhile to record these in your diary for later analysis, but don't let these thoughts destroy your motivation. At the same time that you note these discouraging feelings or experiences, write down a future Proud Line—something you plan to do later that day or early the next day that you'll feel proud about and that will outshine today's gloom.

Sharing your Proud Lines with your weight-watching friends is a good idea. Be sure to validate their Proud Lines. Be careful not to put-down what they feel good about. You can help each other build confidence, trust, self-respect.

CRITERION FOR DETERMINING SUCCESS OF YOUR WEIGHT CONTROL PLAN

You are never really cured of being overweight. The best you can ever hope for is lifetime control. You should measure your success by how long you remain close to your ideal weight. Once you reach your ideal weight, the plan you followed should continue in somewhat modified form as a pattern of life. Hopefully, your weight control plan has reeducated you so that you can maintain a calorie balance without really trying. By the time you reach your ideal weight, counting calories to keep a balance between eating and activity should have become part of your personality.

Granted, you will never be able to go back to your old eating and inactivity patterns without suffering the consequences. However, after several years of continued success the urge to relapse should diminish. It's just not worth risking all you've gained by losing.

Like an alcoholic, you will never be cured. A.A. members are quick to point out that their disease may be under control, but they are still only one drink away from a drunk. Perhaps foodaholics can measure their success the same way. You are never really cured, but after several years of successful calorie-restriction and activity-increase you may consider yourself controlled. But remember—you are only one smorgasbord away from overweight.

Determining
Your Ideal Weight

HEIGHT-WEIGHT BODY FRAME CHARTS

Insurance companies are in the business of life. They know that the longer you live, the longer you pay policy premiums. Therefore, it is to the companies' advantage to keep you alive for as long as possible. The height-weight body frame charts that these companies have published reflect their statistical research findings: the shorter the waist line, the longer the life. One caution: standard height-weight body frame charts, like the Metropolitan Life Insurance Company chart below, have been shown to be approximately 4 to 10 pounds under what a person's ideal weight may really be.[1]

Desirable Weights for Men*

	HEIGHT (with shoes on) 1-inch heels Feet Inches	SMALL FRAME	MEDIUM FRAME	LARGE FRAME
Weight in Pounds According to Frame (In Indoor Clothing)				
Men of Ages 25 and Over	5 2	112–120	118–129	126–141
	5 3	115–123	121–133	129–144
	5 4	118–126	124–136	132–148
	5 5	121–129	127–139	135–152
	5 6	124–133	130–143	138–156
	5 7	128–137	134–147	142–161
	5 8	132–141	138–152	147–166
	5 9	136–145	142–156	151–170
	5 10	140–150	146–160	155–174
	5 11	144–154	150–165	159–179
	6 0	148–158	154–170	164–184
	6 1	152–162	158–175	168–189
	6 2	156–167	162–180	173–194
	6 3	160–171	167–185	178–199
	6 4	164–175	172–190	182–204

* Courtesy of the Metroplitan Life Insurance Company, New York, N. Y.

Desirable Weights for Women*

	HEIGHT (with shoes on) 2-inch heels . Feet Inches	SMALL FRAME	MEDIUM FRAME	LARGE FRAME
Women	4 10	92— 98	96—107	104—119
of Ages 25	4 11	94—101	98—110	106—122
and Over	5 0	96—104	101—113	109—125
	5 1	99—107	104—116	112—128
	5 2	102—110	107—119	115—131
	5 3	105—113	110—122	118—134
	5 4	108—116	113—126	121—138
	5 5	111—119	116—130	125—142
	5 6	114—123	120—135	129—146
	5 7	118—127	124—139	133—150
	5 8	122—131	128—143	137—154
	5 9	126—135	132—147	141—158
	5 10	130—140	136—151	145—163
	5 11	134—144	140—155	149—168
	6 0	138—148	144—159	153—173

For girls between 18 and 25, subtract 1 pound for each year under 25.

Useful as these charts are, they are unfortunately never accompanied by instructions for determining whether you have a large, medium, or small frame. Consequently, most persons incorrectly figure out "Well, I'm such and such a height, and my present weight is within the range of those listed under large frame; therefore, I must have a large frame." Without special anthropometric equipment and testing, your evaluation of your frame size will be nothing more than a guess.

Here are two rules of thumb for more accurately determining your frame size.

1. Circle your wrist with your index finger and thumb. Try as hard as possible to have your thumb and index finger meet or overlap. If they will not meet at all, you have a large frame; if they just barely touch or

* Courtesy of the Metroplitan Life Insurance Company, New York, N. Y.

overlap, you have a medium frame; if your thumb and index finger overlap, you have a small frame.

2. If you are a woman and the circumference of your wrist is 6 inches or less, you have a small frame; if it is between 6 and 6½ inches, your frame is medium; if it is greater than 6½ inches, your frame is large.

    If you are a man, your frame is small if your wrist circumference is less than 6 inches, medium if it is between 6 and 7 inches; and large if it is greater than 7 inches.

The above methods of determining frame size are based on average measurements of thousands of persons. Obviously, there may be special individual differences (like formerly broken wrists or extremely short fingers) that would make for exceptions.

Most people are surprised to find out they are actually one frame size smaller than they thought.

Government statistics on body weights for men and women reflect general averages rather than desired goals. The chart below will not prescribe an ideal weight for you, but at least it shows approximately where you stand in relation to that part of the population that is approximately your age and height.

To interpret this chart, find your height and go across the columns to your present age. Within this area you will see three sets of numbers. Determine the number to which your weight is closest, then note the P-value. This number represents the percentage of the population whose body weight falls below yours. For example, if your body weight is in the column marked P-75, 75% of the people in your height and age categories weigh less than you do. If your weight falls closest to that in the P-50 column, you are average.

MEDIAN AND QUARTILE WEIGHT[1] FOR MEN AND WOMEN, BY AGE AND HEIGHT: UNITED STATES, 1960-62[2]

Ht.	Total, 18-79 years			18-24 years			25-34 years			35-44 years		
	P_{25}	P_{50}	P_{75}	P_{25}	P_{50}	P_{75}	P_{25}	P_{50}	P_{75}	P_{25}	P_{50}	P_{75}

Men — Weight in pounds

Ht.	P_{25}	P_{50}	P_{75}	P_{25}	P_{50}	P_{75}	P_{25}	P_{50}	P_{75}	P_{25}	P_{50}	P_{75}
62"	128	144	164	122	132	175	131	141	152	141	146	152
63"	134	151	163	127	138	162	130	151	158	132	158	178
64"	136	155	167	121	128	156	129	147	163	137	158	167
65"	139	157	177	131	139	159	129	156	174	151	165	183
66"	144	160	177	141	153	170	144	160	174	151	162	180
67"	146	162	180	138	151	168	147	164	187	150	163	178
68"	149	166	185	144	153	168	146	159	182	154	168	184
69"	153	172	187	145	161	184	156	174	188	156	175	189
70"	159	176	195	148	163	177	163	178	196	164	179	195
71"	166	182	201	152	163	177	163	180	200	175	186	204
72"	162	179	198	153	166	183	169	188	208	165	182	197
73"	177	188	208	171	184	195	178	188	206	184	191	202
74"	166	188	209	164	174	207	164	183	201	203	211	215

Women

Ht.	P_{25}	P_{50}	P_{75}	P_{25}	P_{50}	P_{75}	P_{25}	P_{50}	P_{75}	P_{25}	P_{50}	P_{75}
57"	119	130	149	[3]98	[3]116	[3]133	[3]90	[3]112	[3]133	115	125	132
58"	109	129	147	101	107	155	103	110	118	107	118	132
59"	114	130	149	98	112	142	104	118	131	113	128	157
60"	117	133	150	106	117	131	112	123	138	116	132	156
61"	119	137	156	110	121	136	112	120	143	118	130	151
62"	119	136	158	113	125	143	115	127	145	119	135	159
63"	123	137	158	113	122	132	115	128	145	125	138	160
64"	124	138	159	116	126	136	122	133	152	126	140	158
65"	126	139	157	118	132	143	124	134	157	121	137	154
66'	128	140	158	124	137	148	125	136	146	133	142	160
67"	134	152	177	123	134	148	131	147	171	132	150	178
68"	128	147	165	120	129	145	118	147	163	131	148	168

[1]Median—P_{50}, the percentile below which 50 percent of the population fall. Quartiles—P_{25} and P_{75}, the 25th and 75th percentile below which 25 and 75 percent of the population fall.

[2]Height without shoes; weight partially clothed—clothing weight estimated as averaging 2 pounds.

Ht.	45-54 years			55-64 years			65-74 years			75-79 years		
	P_{25}	P_{50}	P_{75}	P_{25}	P_{50}	P_{75}	P_{25}	P_{50}	P_{75}	P_{25}	P_{50}	P_{75}

Men — Weight in pounds

Ht.	P_{25}	P_{50}	P_{75}	P_{25}	P_{50}	P_{75}	P_{25}	P_{50}	P_{75}	P_{25}	P_{50}	P_{75}
62"	131	140	149	115	134	183	155	164	169	122	161	166
63"	137	150	164	140	153	162	140	154	167	126	139	146
64"	150	159	176	141	158	170	142	162	167	129	136	144
65"	143	161	182	137	150	168	137	155	181	140	160	165
66"	148	162	180	145	166	181	137	159	174	138	151	159
67"	151	165	188	148	168	187	141	159	172	145	183	193
68"	153	174	189	153	173	182	147	160	181	163	191	202
69"	153	173	190	161	173	185	141	149	186	138	148	174
70"	164	182	200	151	162	200	166	177	188	[3]156	[3]174	[3]191
71"	174	187	208	166	177	194	157	183	204	[3]162	[3]179	[3]196
72"	170	184	197	162	172	203	[3]159	[3]178	[3]198	[3]167	[3]184	[3]201
73"	167	178	215	205	214	224	[3]162	[3]182	[3]201	[3]172	[3]189	[3]206
74"	150	187	253	[3]171	[3]191	[3]211	[3]166	[3]185	[3]204	[3]177	[3]194	[3]212

Women

Ht.	P_{25}	P_{50}	P_{75}	P_{25}	P_{50}	P_{75}	P_{25}	P_{50}	P_{75}	P_{25}	P_{50}	P_{75}
57"	115	138	166	122	126	130	125	144	150	120	125	130
58"	103	116	130	126	136	148	119	141	159	120	135	163
59"	119	131	148	123	137	149	121	142	160	118	130	146
60"	119	133	150	133	149	165	130	139	154	118	152	162
61"	130	145	166	131	143	162	131	145	162	115	149	183
62"	121	139	159	135	152	178	130	153	172	114	135	154
63"	126	141	160	135	149	180	132	144	163	122	146	156
64"	133	150	176	133	149	176	136	157	174	131	155	191
65"	136	149	177	143	149	184	128	146	157	[3]133	[3]153	[3]173
66"	141	156	175	125	138	165	122	164	182	[3]137	[3]157	[3]176
67"	149	159	179	156	179	186	[3]147	[3]166	[3]185	[3]140	[3]160	[3]180
68"	145	155	170	129	157	180	[3]150	[3]170	[3]189	[3]144	[3]164	[3]183

[3] Estimated values obtained from the linear regression equations.

From U. S. Public Health Service, *Weight, height, and selected body dimensions of adults: United States, 1960-1962.* Washington, D.C.: U. S. Government Printing Office, 1965. Pp. 12-13.

MIRROR TEST

The mirror test is a search for visible fat, bulges, rolls, spare tires, etc. Standing nude in front of a full-length mirror, carefully inspect your body for visible traces of excessive fat. If you look fat in front of a mirror, you probably are fat. Looking in the mirror you can easily discern where you need to reduce as well as where you need to firm up.

How do you feel about the way you look in the mirror? Can you look at yourself and see yourself objectively? Or are you viewing yourself through a distorted carnival fun house mirror? Many dieters have been overweight for so long that their fat image is imbedded in their brain. Even after they do begin to lose weight, they see their old selves whenever they look in the mirror.

If the mirror says you're fat, don't kid yourself—you're fat. But be just as realistic in your self appraisal when the mirror says you're making progress. It may take hours of looking at and studying yourself in front of a mirror, but eventually you will change your self-image and feel good about yourself.

SHIMMY TEST

A variation of the mirror test is the shimmy test. Shake and twist rapidly while standing nude in front of the mirror. If your surface tissue moves in disconcert with the muscle tissues, then you are overweight.

BELTLINE TEST

The beltline test should be used by males only. If your waist measurement at the navel level exceeds your chest measurement at the nipple level, you are overweight. (If the same criterion were used by females, it could indicate either over-weight or flat-chestedness.)

RULER TEST

While lying on your back, place a ruler vertically on your abdomen along the midline of your body. The ruler should touch both the ribs and the pelvic area. If not, you are too fat. The ruler test measures the bulge of the abdominal area. (Therefore it is useless if you are pregnant.)

AGE GAUGE

If you are a man who was satisfied with his weight at age twenty-five, any significant weight gain since that time should be considered excess baggage.

If you are a woman, were you satisfied with your weight at age twenty-one? There is no reason to assume that it is normal to keep gaining weight as you grow older. With care, you can maintain your weight at a steady level, even into middle and advanced age.

PINCH TEST

Approximately fifty percent of all body fat is located just under the skin surface. Average fat deposits are between a quarter of an inch and half an inch thick. The normal skinfold measures between half an inch and one inch. If you pinch yourself and find yourself holding onto more than one inch of fat, you are considered overweight, whatever your body frame size.

Most people distribute fat evenly over their bodies, but

some people seem to accumulate it in certain areas. To determine if your body has a special hiding place for fat, try pinching the following areas: the back of the arm, midway between the shoulder and the elbow; the abdominal area while you are standing (be sure to pull the skin tissue away from the other tissues or muscles of the body); on the back of the calf; at the side of the lower chest, while you are standing. Have someone pinch your back just below your shoulder blade.

If you, or your helper, come up holding significantly more than one inch between thumb and forefinger in any one of the above listed areas, you are overweight.

THE THREE-DOZEN-DOES-IT TEST

Subtract your waist measurement in inches from your height measurement in inches. If the result is 36 or less, you are probably too fat. If it's over 36, you're okay.

This method fails to account for many of the variables related to overweight, such as body frame, or even weight. The simple height-waist ratio is meant to be a quick guide to obesity but may actually be a better test of sagging abdominal muscles.

SURVIVAL TEST

One of the functions of stored fat is to provide potential energy for periods of famine. Using military standards, if an individual can subsist without food for a period of thirty days or more, then the fat reserves within his body were excessive. If the individual could not survive for a period of thirty days, then he was not overweight. (Do not try to use this test to assess your own weight problem. It could prove fatal!)

THE CUBED MIRROR TEST

The cubed mirror test takes into consideration not only the physical aspects of one's ideal weight but also the social aspects. Your ideal weight is the weight at which you:

1. Feel best   a. To yourself
2. Look best   b. To members of
                        the same sex
3. Act best   c. To members of
                        the opposite sex

After you have used the Mirror Test to make your own judgment about your ideal weight, solicit the opinions of several members of both sexes. Remember to tell them to consider not only how you look to them, but also how you feel, and act, as they see it.

Sometimes we look okay at a particular weight and yet "feel" heavy. Friends of the same sex will probably give you their honest opinions. However, most women believe you can't be too thin. This high-fashion thinness is not necessarily what most males desire. Among certain African tribes, seatoplegia—having a big rump—is highly prized. The woman with the biggest rump, which is often shaped with baling wire, is considered the most beautiful in the tribe. Don't take off for Africa. Somewhere in between England's Twiggy and Africa's seatoplegiac there exists, no doubt, a realistic balance.

INTERPRETING OVERWEIGHT

No one method of determining your ideal weight is so accurate that it should be taken as the final word. Using some criteria, many people whose weight falls within normal limits could be considered overweight, or even obese, at different points in their lives. Most well-trained athletes are overweight according to the criteria of height-weight body frame charts. Therefore, the Public Health Service has cautioned:

> *It cannot be overstressed that assigning a label of obese to any one person or group of persons should come only after a comprehensive assessment of all pertinent factors. The sex of the subject, age, body type, and state of health, along with specific measurements such as skinfold thickness, must be considered in determining if a person is obese. Comparing any individual or group in terms of their heights and weights with a given set of averages or standards does not give adequate information on which to assess obesity since such comparisons imply weight not fatness.[2]*

Here is a good rule of thumb: If you failed three or more of the above tests, chances are good that you are not at your ideal weight.

SCIENTIFIC METHODS

Scientific methods of determining one's degree of overweight are generally not practical for measuring large segments of the population. But two of these methods should be mentioned because of their accuracy in assessing ideal weight.

The Densimetric method is based on the principle that body fat weighs less (is less dense) than lean mass tissue, which is primarily composed of bone and muscle. Using water as the standard, a given amount of fat weighs less than the same amount of water. Bone and muscle tissue weigh more than water. The greater the amount of fat in a person's body, the more buoyant he is—that is, the easier it is for him to float in water. Well-trained athletes, whose percentage of body fat is low and whose muscular systems are highly developed, generally cannot float. Even when they expand their lungs to their fullest capacity, athletes are incapable of displacing enough water to float.

Determining ideal weight by the Densimetric Method involves three steps. First the subject is weighed. Then he is instructed to inhale deeply, filling his lungs to their greatest capacity. Holding his breath, he is weighed under water. Finally, he is brought out of the water and the volume of air he has been holding in his lungs is measured.

All three of these variables—weight, underwater weight, and the volume of air held in the lungs are plugged into a formula with several constants in order to determine the subject's total percentage of body fat.

Hydrometry is a method of determining the total body water retained by an individual. Since it is known that fat is approximately 30% water, one can determine the amount of fat contained within a person's body. The method is simple. A chemical injected into the body will be diluted to a greater degree in the body of a fatter individual. By measuring the concentration of this chemical, one can accurately assess the amount of water being retained.

BODY IMAGE VERSUS BODY REALITY

What you see is not always what you are. Overweight individuals often view themselves through distorted glasses. This distortion can work in several ways. Sometimes the over-weight person may see himself as heavier than he really is. When he looks into a mirror, he sees a bigger abdominal cavity, larger buttocks and huge thighs. This self-image is difficult to shake, even if the person's weight actually decreases markedly.

Other overweight people see themselves as much slimmer than they really are. These are the people who often rationalize away their need for weight control programs.

And some people manage to see their bodies as they really are.

Those with realistic body concepts tend to have the greatest success in their weight control programs, because dieters must continually reassess their body image as they lose weight.

Nothing could be more devastating to an individual whose scale says he has lost a significant amount of weight than looking into the mirror and seeing his old, fat self. This individual can only see himself as fat. Yet most weight control plans fail to consider this important psychological mechanism of self-perception.

Few successful dieters actually see themselves as thin, especially when they first reach their ideal weight. Only after months of living a thin life does the successful dieter begin to feel good about himself. Once he has reached his ideal weight, the individual must take time to enjoy himself and rediscover his own beauty. He must study himself in front of a mirror, and not be afraid to love himself.

REFERENCES

1. Mayer, Jean, *Overweight,* Englewood Cliffs, N. J.: Prentice-Hall, Inc., 1968, p. 28.

2. U. S. Public Health Service. *Obesity and Health,* Washington, D. C.: U. S. Government Printing Office, no date; p. 2.

You Are What You Eat

"You are what you eat"
Said a wise old man.
And Lord if that's true
I'm a garbage can.

VICTOR BUONO[1]

    If people really were what they ate, then they might look like   hamburgerfrenchfrypotatochipicecreamhotdogchocolatecakepopcornpizzapickle people.

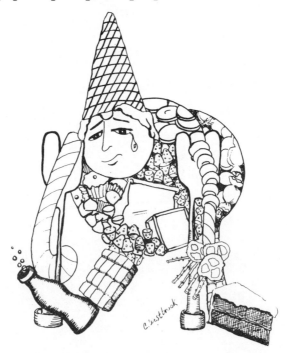

However, thanks to our genetic code, our bodies utilize the nutrients from these various foodstuffs, and rebuild them according to their DNA blueprints. Biochemically speaking, then, what you eat today will walk and talk tomorrow.

Your body requires approximately 55 nutrients. These nutrients must be consumed on a regular basis, especially while you are restricting your calorie intake, if your system is to function efficiently and comfortably.

Even while on a diet, you can consume all of these necessary nutrients without too much hassle. And if you're among the many dieters who are interested in their appearance, paying attention to nutrients will pay off. Disregarding nutritional requirements works *against* your appearance in subtle ways. A diet devoid of fresh fruits and vegetables, for example, may cost you the clear skin, bright eyes, and healthy hair you've always prided yourself on.

So, while you're cutting down on the quantity of food you eat, make sure what you do eat contains enough of the right elements. Overfed people are generally over-weight. But overweight people can actually be malnourished because of the low-nutrient foods they choose to consume.

OUR 38,000 HOUR HABIT

If it takes you thirty minutes to finish each meal you eat, then you spend approximately one-and-a-half hours eating each day. Time spent in planning, shopping, preparing the food and cleaning up after meals is considerably more. And don't forget the time consumed in coffee breaks, parties, or midnight snacks, as well as the time spent just *thinking* about food.

Adding it all up, it seems reasonable to say that by the time you reach the age of seventy, you will have devoted over 38,000 hours of your life—and, conservatively, about $50,000—to food.

Your dietary habits play a very important role in determining the condition of your health, the size of your pocketbook and the way you spend your time. Yet, it is appalling to think of the numbers of Americans who are poorly informed about the science of nutrition. One would think that the amount of time and money we spend eating proportionately reflect our knowledge and practices about nutrition. On the contrary, our feeding behavior only reveals the depth of our ignorance.

Most people are not in the habit of talking about the nutritional aspects of food. Perhaps this is because eating— like making love—is one thing most people would rather do than talk about. Just as a child picks up negative, nonverbal information about sexuality, so does he unconsciously learn about nutrition, absorbing the misinformation and misconceptions of his elders. It seems ironic that in our enlightened society children grow up with a high degree of ignorance in these two important areas.

These children will become adults and, eventually, parents. Unless considerable amounts of time and effort are spent to improve their nutritional knowledge, the cycle of ignorance will be perpetuated. The misconceptions that have been passed down have produced a generation of Americans whose nutritional practices blatantly oppose what is known to be true and healthful.

Nutritional ignorance is not limited to any particular economic or ethnic group. Most people suffer from intellectual retardation regarding nutrition, having an almost total lack of any functional knowledge. Surprising as it may seem, most people know no more about nutrition as full-grown adults than they did as breastfeeding infants.

It would seem logical that if we spend so much time, energy and money on eating, the prudent individual would willingly devote an appropriate number of hours to learning about nutrition. If this were done, the basic level of knowledge accumulated could make a significant contribution to his health for the rest of his life.

Any interested individual could inform himself through a personally-motivated reading program, or by taking an adult education course. But, ideally, nutrition information should be taught as part of a sound health education program, so that most people would be exposed to it during their earlier years of formal education.

WHERE DID WE GO WRONG?

For the most part, we have not been taught but have simply inferred most of our nutritional ideas. To see how much of our nutritional knowledge is inferred, let's look back to our early childhood. No child escapes nutrition education. From our first sucking at mother's breast, to observing mother's wrinkled-up nose at the smell of certain baby foods, to watching father lick his plate clean, every child receives nutrition education. Unfortunately it often comes in the form of negative, nonverbal learning. Dr. Charles Galloway, an expert in nonverbal communication, suggests that nonverbal communication is the primary avenue through which children learn, especially before they themselves can communicate verbally.[2]

Research concerning nonverbal behavior implies that when a discrepancy exists between verbal and nonverbal signals, the child will usually believe the nonverbal. For example, most children are encouraged or required to eat vegetables at dinner. Yet, too often, they observe that their parents do not even put vegetables on their own plates. This nonverbal behavior message speaks louder than their parents' words, and it is this behavior that the child grasps and probably imitates. The child has indeed been educated; he has learned, but not in a manner conducive to the formation of healthy lifetime nutrition patterns.

THE ILTEN SIGN

The nutritional messages taught in the home often carry a negative tone. This negative learning has a lasting effect. Let us imagine that from birth until death we all wear an ILTEN sign—an acronym for "I Love To Eat Nutritiously." As a child progresses through each day, and accumulates negative experiences in relation to nutrition, parts of his ILTEN sign are ripped off. As time passes, this sign is slowly mutilated, until by the adolescent years very little of the original sign remains intact.

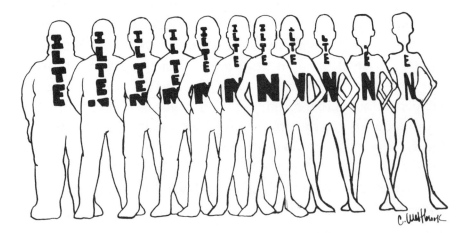

Letters of the ILTEN sign can drip off at either end. If, for example, parents apply pressure through the "eat or else approach"—or else: no dessert, no T.V., early to bed—little pieces of the sign begin to rip off at the "IL" end.

The "I Love" end of the sign is also damaged when bickering occurs during mealtime; when cold or quickie meals are served; when meals are eaten alone; when meals are hurried; when parents are overly concerned about manners and neatness; or at any other time when eating does not prove to be an enjoyable experience.

The "Nutrition" end of the sign begins to shred when children are served unbalanced meals; when there is little variety or selection; when children register the nonverbal information that parents eat only what they want to eat, but force their children to eat what they should eat; when children are permitted to choose their own snacks without supervision; when children are bombarded by exposure to junk food advertisements; or in any other situation that conditions the child away from well-balanced, sensible eating patterns.

Once either or both ends of the sign are destroyed, nothing short of massive nutritional reeducation can repair the damage.

1. Was your ILTEN sign ever ripped? From which end?

2. Relate some specific incidents that illustrate this.

3. List several ways that the dieter can begin to develop nutritional eating patterns that restore the love for eating.

4.   How can you as a dieter repair your torn ILTEN sign?

DIETARY SELF-ANALYSIS

One of the best ways to repair torn ILTEN signs is to take time for introspective examination of your dietary habits. You may begin to recognize practices of which you may never have been aware.

Complete the following strategies in writing as honestly as you can. Don't be frightened by your responses. Your goal is to learn something about your life experiences that will provide some insight into your nutritional practices. Writing is a very important complement to introspection. Avoid the temptation to just think through these exercises. Be conscientious in completing each one in writing.

Philosophy of Eating Continuum

Socrates once said, "Bad men live that they may eat and drink, whereas good men eat and drink that they might live." He was making a value judgment that reflected his philosophy of eating.

Where do you find yourself on the continuum below? Are you the type of person who plans your day around food, and thinks food around the clock? Or, perhaps you're the person who looks at his watch and says, "My, it's 2:30 P.M. and I haven't had a thing to eat all day."

Write your initials at the point on the continuum where you belong right now. Print your name where you would like to be.

Write an "I realize . . . " or "I will . . . " sentence describing your reaction to the continuum. Think about your feelings about your philosophy of eating, especially as it affects your weight control plan.

Philosophy of Eating Continuum

LIVE-TO-EAT :   :   :   : XXXX :   :   :   : EAT-TO-LIVE
      LIEF   ERIC

Open comment:

Ten Foods I Love Most to Eat and Drink

In the chart provided below, list your ten favorite foods. Be sure to include foods that you may only eat on special occasions such as birthdays, or during certain seasons of the year. Enter the date on which you last had this food.

Put checks in the appropriate columns using the following codings:

FAVORITE FOODS

A   Food you prefer to eat or drink when alone
+   Relatively high in nutrients
-    High in calories and low in nutrients—junk foods
*   Low in calories
#   Food that you eat too much of and/or too often
¢   Costs under 50¢ a portion

$ Costs more than one dollar a portion
5   Would not have been on your list 5 years ago
☺   Food that you feel happy just thinking about
!   Food you plan to cut out during your diet
TV   Food you eat while watching TV
:   Food you plan to eat smaller portions of during your diet

Favorite Foods	Date	A	+	–	*	#	¢	$	5	☺	!	TV	:
1.													
2.													
3.													
4.													
5.													
6.													
7.													
8.													
9.													
10.													

Objectively study the coding, just as a scientist would interpret data. Look for patterns you may not have been aware of before. For example, are the junk foods also the foods you eat when you're alone in front of the TV?

1. What did the Ten Favorite Foods exercise reveal to you about your food selection?

2. What, if anything, do you plan to *do* about your diet as a result of this exercise?

Value Voting

This strategy asks you, on the one hand, to acknowledge what you believe and how strongly you believe it; and, on the other hand, to indicate how strongly you are committed to your belief in terms of your actual behavior.

To the left of each statement you will find the following scale. Circle the response which best represents what you *think*.

SA = Strongly Agree
A = Agree
N = Neutral, Do Not Agree or Disagree
D = Disagree
SD = Strongly Disagree

To the right of each statement is the following scale. Circle the response that most closely tells what you *do* in relation to the statement.

A = Always
F = Frequently
S = Sometimes
R = Rarely
N = Never

SA A N D SD	I should take large doses of Vitamin C to prevent or cure a cold.	A F S R N
SA A N D SD	I should take daily Vitamin A supplements.	A F S R N
SA A N D SD	I should drink at least three glasses of milk a day.	A F S R N
SA A N D SD	Increasing my activity would be beneficial to my weight reduction program.	A F S R N
SA A N D SD	I should engage in some vigorous activity three times or more per week.	A F S R N
SA A N D SD	Consuming large quantitites of sugar may lead to heart disease.	A F S R N
SA A N D SD	Snacking on pizza is okay.	A F S R N
SA A N D SD	Snacking on chocolate is bad.	A F S R N
SA A N D SD	Keep away from potatoes if you're dieting.	A F S R N
SA A N D SD	I need to do something about my weight.	A F S R N
SA A N D SD	Snacking on potato chips can ruin a diet.	A F S R N
SA A N D SD	It's all right to drink one sugar-containing soft drink a day.	A F S R N
SA A N D SD	I should drink skim milk.	A F S R N
SA A N D SD	I can consume ice cream regularly.	A F S R N
SA A N D SD	I should use weight reduction pills.	A F S R N
SA A N D SD	I should follow the ideas in this book.	A F S R N
SA A N D SD	I should approve of myself.	A F S R N

SA A N D SD	I should go to a profit-making organization for assistance.	A F S R N
SA A N D SD	I will reach my goal weight.	A F S R N
SA A N D SD	I can maintain my goal weight.	A F S R N
SA A N D SD	I should not believe food advertisements.	A F S R N
SA A N D SD	I should allow advertisements to influence my buying.	A F S R N
SA A N D SD	I should use nationally advertised brand-name products.	A F S R N

Examine your responses to the statements. See if you can detect any patterns. Write a comment in the space below concerning the general strength of your beliefs and about the consistency or inconsistency between your beliefs and your practices. For example, perhaps you learned that, even though you believe vigorous activity is very important, you don't actually engage in it three or more times a week.

Perhaps you will discover that the preponderance of your responses were neutral. If you do not strongly agree or strongly disagree with anything, is it possible that you lack knowledge about these issues? Could your lack of strong convictions explain your previous failures at weight control?

Open Comments: _____

_____

_____

Rank Ordering

This self-evaluation technique attempts to establish priorities. Priorities often reveal values. At different points in our lives we need to take the time to examine, rearrange, and reorder our priorities. New information, different beliefs, new experiences, and unusual circumstances create the need to reexamine former values.

Rank order from one to four the following groups of alternatives. Write number one next to the choice that you rank highest in the category and write number four next to the choice that you rank lowest.

1. Rank in order of nutrition value:

    _____ Instant Breakfast with water
    _____ salted peanuts
    _____ pizza with pepperoni
    _____ orange drink with a B-complex vitamin
             pill

2. Rank as sources of nutrition information:

    _____ nutritionists
    _____ a diet book author
    _____ a medical doctor
    _____ a newspaper article

3. Rank as reliable sources of weight control information:

    _____ a dietician
    _____ a "fat" doctor
    _____ a magazine ad
    _____ a pharmacist

4. Rank in order of your choice from a vending machine:

_____ a chocolate bar
_____ a box of raisins
_____ a pack of chewing gum
_____ a chocolate bar with nuts

5. Re-rank the same items in order of nutrition value:

_____ a chocolate bar
_____ a box of raisins
_____ a pack of chewing gum
_____ a chocolate bar with nuts

6. Rank your meals in order of preference:

_____ Breakfast
_____ Lunch
_____ Dinner
_____ Snacks

Answers to the rankings that are matters of fact:

1. 4,2,1,3
5. 3,2,4,1

REFERENCES

1. Buono, V. *"Fat Man's Prayer,"* from an album entitled: *Heavy*! Dore Records, 1608 Argle, Hollywood, California.
2. Galloway, Charles M., "The Challenge of Nonverbal Research," *Theory Into Practice*, Vol. 10, No. 4 (October, 1971), pp. 310-314. Also: C. M. Galloway, "Nonverbal: The Language of Sensitivity," *Theory Into Practice*, Vol. 10, No.4, pp. 227-230.

A Little Nutrition With Your Weight Control Please!

Too many of today's popular weight control schemes are concerned only with the shedding of pounds. If you plan to be on a reduced calorie-intake plan for longer than several weeks, you should be aware of the nutritional value of your weight control plan.

An alcoholic can try to avoid booze completely. A heroin addict can try to remove himself completely from the drug environment. But the weight watcher can neither completely avoid food, nor completely remove himself from an environment where food is present. He must eat to live. Being exposed to just a little food often triggers the sort of response that would send an alcoholic or an addict on a month-long binge.

Herein lies the dilemma of the American dieter: "How do I stop when I've had enough? Once I've had enough, how do I keep from having too much—even of good nutritious food?"

Knowledge alone does not usually produce behavior change. However, once we have determined to change our behavior we need information to help us make rational choices. We need knowledge in order to formulate the values that will guide our lives.

Even the most enthusiastic calorie-conscious dieter may overlook some basic nutritional concepts. A reduction in caloric intake generally reduces the total amount of food an individual consumes. Unless he carefully considers the nutrient content of the foods he does eat, the dieter may easily cheat his body of essential nutrients. The desire to look slim and attractive can often backfire if nutrients are as severely restricted as calories.

Please, add a little nutrition to your weight control!

Nutritional deficiencies, combined with calorie restriction, can cause fatigue and a general run-down feeling. This feeling in turn depletes your zest and enthusiasm for your weight control program and before you know it, you're off again on the dangerous cycle of yo-yo dieting. If you are informed about the interrelations among nutrition, calories, activity, and behavior, you will be able to sustain a quiet, steady motivation that will endure through the traumas of losing weight. Some of the more revolutionary plans generate fire-ball enthusiasm as they motivate you to burn up large fat reserves. What actually happens on quick weight loss plans is that there is a significant loss of protein and of large quantities of water—not a healthy approach for sustained dieting. Usually motivation to pursue such plans also burns out quickly. Perhaps this is nature's method of self-preservation, since prolonged adherence to these poorly-balanced diets would be hazardous to your health.

SHORTCOMINGS OF THE AMERICAN DIET

While it is difficult to generalize about nutritional deficiencies in the American diet, recent studies indicate certain trends in the diet of groups studied. A ten-state cross-cultural, cross-ethnic, cross-age, sex, and geographic location nutritional survey conducted by the Department of Health, Education, and Welfare indicated that a significant percentage of the population studied manifested some nutritional difficulties, including malnutrition. Iron deficiency was found throughout, but was most severe in low income Black males and females.[1]

Most American dietary surveys show that the following nutrients are frequently deficient in the diets of most age groups; *calcium, vitamin A, iron* (in women), and *vitamin C.*

Calcium is by far the most abundant mineral element in the body. About 99% of this mineral is concentrated in the bones and teeth. Calcium combines with other minerals to help give the skeletal system its strength.

Dairy products account for approximately three-fourths of the calcium in the average American diet. If on your diet you are avoiding milk, cheese, yogurt, or ice cream, you would require a high intake of foods such as collards, turnip greens, mustard greens, kale, clams, oysters, broccoli, or shrimp in order to fulfill the recommended adult requirement of 800 milligrams of calcium per day. Even on a restricted calorie intake, milk products should not be entirely omitted from the diet since they provide calcium, as well as many other essential and worthwhile nutrients.

Vitamin A is needed in only very small amounts. Large amounts of this vitamin can be stored in the liver and in fat tissues, so a daily intake is not really necessary. Vitamin A helps your eyes maintain normal vision in dim light. It also contributes to the quality of skin tissue, and appears to be important in the skeletal growth and the tooth structure during the early developmental years.

A deficiency in this nutrient may manifest itself in poor skin and hair quality. Or you may experience extreme difficulty seeing in the dark, especially right after a bright light shines in your eyes. Night blindness, medically called nyctalopia, may contribute to a significant number of nighttime automobile accidents.

Vitamin A is found in two forms. Pure vitamin A in concentrated amounts comes from foods such as fish, liver and oils. Milk, butter, fortified margarine, cheese, and egg yolks also contain large amounts of vitamin A. Carotenes are another form of vitamin A, and they are available in green or deep yellow vegetable plants. Abundant quantities of carotene are found in spinach, turnip tops, beet greens, asparagus, broccoli, carrots, sweet potatoes, winter squash, pumpkin, apricots, peaches, and cantaloupe. Generally, the darker the color of the plant, the more carotene contained therein. When we discard the green outer leaves of lettuce and eat the colorless leaves, we throw away significant amounts of vitamin A.

Lack of *iron* is another shortcoming in the American diet, particularly among teen-age girls and pregnant or lactating women. Although the total amount of iron in the body is only about 5 grams, its function is extremely important. Iron is a basic constituent of hemoglobin, which combines with oxygen and is carried to the tissues for cell metabolism. Even though the body conserves much of its iron stores, a woman may suffer from iron deficiency anemia if, in her childbearing years, she does not eat foods rich in this nutrient. Amenorrhea (missed periods) or scanty menstruation can be due to inadequate intake of iron.

Dairy products are a poor source of iron. Mothers, particularly nursing mothers, must take care to introduce their infants to iron-rich foods early in life.

Liver is an excellent source of iron, and so are other organ meats, lean meats, shellfish, and egg yolks. Baked beans are a good source of iron, as are certain fruits such as peaches, apricots, prunes, grapes, and raisins. Enriched breads and cereals also provide a significant amount of iron.

Interestingly enough, in the past a regular supply of dietary iron came from water running through iron pipes and from cooking in iron pots. Modern "improved" aluminum materials have eliminated this source, so it is now necessary to more carefully select iron-rich foods.[2]

The following list should provide you with many choices of iron-rich sources, particularly for your snacks. If you are deficient in iron (and many people are), your blood lacks sufficient oxygen to burn up calories for needed energy. This accounts for the tired, rundown feeling you experience. A prudent selection of iron-rich snack foods—raisins, prunes, apricots, nuts, peanut butter, figs, grapes, dates—will help alleviate that feeling. (If you are concerned about the effects on your teeth of the natural sugar contained in dried fruits, it would be advisable to brush your teeth after snacking on dried fruits.)

Foods High in Iron*

Food	Serving	Mg. iron
Apricots, dried	5 halves	1.5
Bitter chocolate	1 square	1.3
Clams	2 oz.	4.2
Dandelion greens	1/2 cup	2.3
Dates	3, 4	.6
Egg	1	1.4
Figs, dried	2	.9
Ham, smoked	2 oz.	1.7
Hazelnuts	10-12	.6
Kale	3/4 cup	1.7
Kidney beef	2 oz.	4.7
Lamb, leg	2 oz.	1.9
Lentils	1/2 cup cooked	2.2

*Adapted from: Mayo Clinic Diet Manual, 3rd edition. Philadelphia: W. B. Saunders Company, 1961, pp. 188-189.

Liver, beef	2 oz.	4.7
Oatmeal	1/2 cup cooked	.7
Oysters, raw	2 oz.	3.4
Parsley	10 sprigs	.4
Peaches, dried	1 1/2	1.9
Popcorn	1 cup popped	.4
Pork loin	2 oz.	1.8
Prunes, dried	4	1.2
Raisins, dried	5 tb.	1.7
Sardines	2 oz.	1.6
Shrimp, canned	2 oz.	1.9
Soybeans, dried	2 tb.	2.0
Spinach	1/2 cup cooked	1.5
Tongue, beef	2 oz.	1.7
Turkey	2 oz.	2.3
Turnip greens	1/2 cup	1.8
Veal roast	2 oz.	2.2
Walnuts	8-15 halves	.3
Wheat, shredded	1 biscuit	1.1

Vitamin C—ascorbic acid—is another nutrient frequently neglected in the American diet. Vitamin C helps protect the body against infection, but this should not be confused with preventing or curing the common cold, despite the claims of many well-intentioned writers. This fresh-food vitamin is found in its highest concentration in the fruit and juices of oranges, grapefruit, lemons, limes, fresh strawberries, cantaloupe, and pineapple. Tomatoes and certain nonacidic fresh fruits are also sources of vitamin C—peaches, pears, apples, bananas, blueberries, and watermelon. Certain vegetables like broccoli, Brussels sprouts, spinach, kale, green peppers, cabbage, and even potatoes (white or sweet) considerably enhance one's vitamin C intake.

Perhaps the most logical way to insure a proper daily vitamin C intake is to have an orange or orange juice, grapefruit, or grapefruit juice for breakfast. Since many Americans skip breakfast, this may in part explain why ascorbic acid is one of the nutrients in limited supply in our diets.

BREAK(THE)FAST

I know that three meals a day is the healthy way,
but I can't eat breakfast on an empty stomach!

SANDRA WEINER, STUDENT
TOWSON STATE COLLEGE

Confirmed non-breakfast-eaters say things like, "But I don't have time to eat breakfast in the morning;" or "It makes me nauseous just to think about food so early;" or "I'm not hungry in the morning so I might just as well save calories then." If you are a non-breakfast-eater, it is possible that your food chart will reveal that your snacking pattern has you consuming as many calories during a coffee and doughnut break as you might have had in a well-balanced breakfast.

A substantial breakfast provides one-quarter of the day's nutrients, including proteins, fats, minerals, carbohydrates, and vitamins. A continental breakfast does not supply one-fourth of the day's needed nutrients.

If you experience a midmorning drag somewhere between the hours of nine and noon, this sag in efficiency and pep may have a nutritional origin. You usually finish your last meal around seven or eight in the evening. If you were to eat breakfast at seven or eight the next morning, you would be breaking a twelve-hour fast, assuming, of course, that you had had no midnight snack before retiring.

The liver can only store about a twelve-hour supply of sugar, and the blood carries a two-to-three hour supply. Breakfast is a convenient time to resupply and supplement the liver's fast-depleting supply of this source of stored energy. By skipping breakfast, you extend the normal twelve-hour fast, thereby causing a net blood sugar deficiency for about one to two hours. When the blood sugar and liver sugar supplies are both depleted, you are likely to feel fatigue. This usually occurs just before lunch.

Furthermore, if there are great physical demands, an individual with an empty stomach will more quickly deplete the liver's supply of glycogen. Physical exertion without an adequate breakfast may cause you to feel dizzy, weak, or even to pass out. If you have noticed this drag, you are probably putting an unnecessary strain on your system by asking your body to extend its normal nightly fast. The brain and nervous system can only function when there is an adequate supply of glucose or blood sugar. If your "get up and go" feels like it got up and went, your central nervous system may be trying to tell you something.

Where do you fit on the Breakfast Continuum? Write your initials where appropriate. Write your name where you would *like* to be.

Breakfast Continuum

INDISCRIMINATE BREAKFASTER INA— EATS VORACIOUSLY   :   :   :   :   **XXXX**   :   :   :   : BREAKFAST DECLINER BRENDA— BECOMES QUEASY AT THE THOUGHT OF FOOD BEFORE NOON.

Open comment:

If you have been skipping breakfast, it may take several weeks to adjust to a changed routine, but the rewards in increased efficiency will be well worth the effort. Lack of time is a poor excuse. If you enjoy sleeping until the last possible moment, you can still manage to eat an adequate breakfast in less than five minutes by freezing French toast, eggs, or waffles ahead of time in large quantities. While you pop your daily portion into the oven to heat, you can attend to your normal morning routines.

PRAGMATIC NUTRITION

In response to the need for a simple way to deal with human nutrition, the Institute of Home Economics, United States Department of Agriculture, developed categories known as the Four Food Groups.

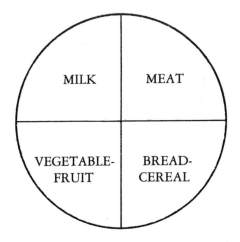

The following chart will tell you how many servings from each of the four groups an adequate daily diet should contain.

Four Food Groups—

MILK GROUP

Two or more servings daily for the adult.
(Children and pregnant women 3 or more servings; teenagers and nursing women 4 or more servings.)

One serving:

Milk: 1 cup (8 ounces)

Cheese: 1 ounce

Yogurt: 1 cup

Ice Cream: 1 pint (16 ounces)

VEGETABLE-FRUIT GROUP

Four or more servings (including requirements for vitamins C and A).

One serving: ½ cup or 4 ounces of fruits and vegetables.

One daily serving of vitamin C from—

Citrus fruit	Cabbage
Strawberries	Potato
Cantaloupe	Salad greens
Tomato	

Every-other-day serving of vitamin A from—

Dark green or deep yellow vegetables: peppers, broccoli, asparagus, squash, pumpkin, etc.

Daily Food Guide

MEAT GROUP

Two or more servings daily.

One serving:
> Poultry, fish, lean cooked beef, veal, pork, lamb:
> 2 to 3 ounces

> Eggs: 2

> Beans, peas, lentils: 1 cup cooked dry

> Peanut butter: 4 tablespoons

BREAD-CEREAL GROUP

Four or more servings daily.

One serving:
> Bread (whole grain, enriched, or restored): 1 slice

> Ready-to-eat cereal: 1 ounce

> Cooked cereal, corn meal, grits, macaroni, noodles,
> rice, spaghetti: ½ to ¾ cup.

This Daily Food Guide allows for considerable flexibility in food selection. Variety and moderation should be your guiding principles as you select foods from each group. Variety of texture and color in foods, varied methods of preparation, and the selection of various ethnic delicacies contribute to a well-balanced diet and minimize the "food blahs." Food is more than just something to eat!

When consumed in large quantitites or too frequently, even good foods can become detrimental to your health. Eggs, for example, are an excellent source of many nutrients, but if you had as many as five per day you could significantly detract from their beneficial qualities because you would limit selection of foods containing other necessary nutrients.

It's the quality of the food, moderated by the quantity, and spiced by variety that makes for sensible nutrition. As rich in certain nutrients as milk is, two quarts of whole milk per day would provide 1,320 calories. This would occupy slots in your diet that could be better filled with foods providing the nutrients that milk lacks.

The Four Food Groups form your nutritional foundation. Selecting foods as recommended in these groupings utilizes approximately half of the calories required by an adult, while providing all of the protein, vitamin A, vitamin B_2 (riboflavin), vitamin C (ascorbic acid), and calcium necessary to maintain health. Nearly all of the B_1 (thiamin) and niacin will also be supplied.

The greatest deficiency of this guide is that it provides only about one-half of the RDA iron content for women in their childbearing years. Nevertheless, it provides an excellent set of guidelines as we begin to travel down the road of proper nutrition. We can build on this Four Food Group foundation by supplementing our diets with foods rich in iron or in whatever nutrients we need.

It is a good idea to bear in mind the Four Food Groups as we plan our meals, and especially when we select our snack foods. Two groups of foods not included in the Four Food Groups are junk foods consisting mostly of "empty calories," such as potato chips, pretzels, candy, soft drinks, alcoholic beverages, sugar; and miscellaneous foods like coffee, tea, condiments, spices, artificial sweeteners. The miscellaneous group adds significantly to the overall palatability of the diet without adding significantly to the calories, but neither of these groupings provides significant nutrients in relation to your total daily needs. A good rule of thumb to use when selecting foods is: do the calories exceed the nutritive value?

Although the Four Food Groups Guide has been criticized for not meeting all of our nutritional needs, it has the distinct advantage of reducing a very complex biochemical science to a simple practical system that can be understood and remembered. Without restricting your food selection, this approach classifies foods into a practical system which balances almost all of the 55 nutrients needed to maintain your health.

MILK GROUP

Cheese, ice cream, yogurt, and milk comprise this food group. Many important nutrients such as calcium, riboflavin, protein, and other minerals and vitamins are found within this group in appreciable amounts.

However, it is important to point out that there is more to good nutrition than just drinking milk. There is no perfect food, not even a "nearly perfect" food. Sometimes a milk lover will fill himself up with milk and crowd out many other good foods. Often children drink their milk before eating and then claim they are too full to eat the meal. However, by the time dessert is served, they claim they're hungry! They are not lying. The fact is this perfect timing occurs because the all-liquid diet moves out of the stomach in five to fifteen minutes—which correlates nicely with dessert time.

Recently there has been some investigation of a possible lack of tolerance to lactose (milk sugar) among Greeks, Arabs, Jews, Blacks, Japanese, and Filipinos.[3] It appears that certain ethnic groups, who may not be accustomed to lactose, lack the digestive enzyme—lactase—that normally helps metabolize the milk sugar, lactose. Without lactase, lactose will not be digested properly, producing certain clinical manifestations that may include flatulence, bloating, abdominal pain, and diarrhea.

However, in some of the studies large quantities of lactose were administered to individuals who were unaccustomed to consuming lactose. Under those conditions, most people would be lactose-intolerant. Perhaps small quantities of milk given gradually over time would allow the system to develop the necessary lactase to metabolize the lactose. Certain cheeses not containing lactose are better tolerated than milk or ice cream. There is still much to be learned about lactose intolerance, and it is not suggested that people completely eliminate milk products from their diets. Milk supplies approximately three-fourths of our daily calcium requirement.

Identify where you fit on the Milk Group Continuum. The middle represents someone who follows the recommendations of the Four Food Groups.

Milk Group Continuum

MILK-SATURATED :   :   :   : **XXXX** :   :   :   : LACTOSE-LIMITED
MIKE   LUKE

Open comment:

The following chart suggests the quantity of other calcium-containing foods that would have to be consumed to equal one serving, or eight ounces, of milk.

CALCIUM EQUIVALENTS OF
EIGHT OUNCES OF MILK

1½ oz. cheese

12 oz. of ice cream

12 oz. cottage cheese

3⅝ lbs. carrots

3⅜ lbs. cabbage

12 eggs

5 large grapefruit

6 oranges

10 lbs. potatoes

½ to ¾ lbs. of kale, turnip, or mustard greens

2 lbs. broccoli

¾ lb endive

2 lbs. cooked green beans

4 lbs. green peas

In choosing milk and milk products and their alternatives, you may want to consider, in addition to the calcium content, the price and the calories.

Skim milk	90 calories
1% butterfat milk	115 "
2% butterfat milk	137 "
Whole milk, 3.5% butterfat	165 "

MEAT GROUP

The foods in the meat group provide the bulk of high-quality protein. Protein molecules are made up of smaller building blocks called amino acids. There are 22 amino acids, eight of which are *essential* for adults, and nine, possibly ten, of which are needed by infants and children during growth spurts. An essential amino acid is one that the body cannot synthesize or manufacture from its basic chemicals. A *complete* protein provides the individual with all eight of the essential amino acids. These eight essential amino acids must be supplied directly from the diet if normal growth and development are to take place.

Lean cooked beef, veal, lamb, pork, poultry, and fish are all concentrated sources of complete protein. But meat sources are also the most expensive sources, and also the highest in calories per serving. Muscle fibers of meat are laced with fat particles, the most concentrated source of calories. If you eat enormous servings of meat daily, excessive protein calories will make you just as fat as excessive carbohydrate or starch calories.

In order to keep the calories, and, amid rapidly rising food prices, the grocery bill, down you might wish to consider alternative sources of the essential amino acids. Beans, dried peas, lentils, and nuts, including peanut butter, can function in combination to fulfill the necessary protein requirements. Two eggs constitute a serving of high quality protein.

Americans generally consume excessive quantities of meat. Currently a movement to minimize meat consumption is having an impact on our country.[4] Proponents of this movement suggest that many of earth's labors are squandered. To provide prime meats we feed our cows grain that could be feeding our human populations. Grain fed cattle may consume as much as twenty pounds of grain for each pound of edible return. Conversion of grains into meat through a rudiment system is inefficient. With four stomachs, the cow can easily convert non-humanly edible substances, such as grass, into meat.

VEGETABLE-FRUIT GROUP

Within the four daily servings recommended from the Vegetable and Fruit Group, this group has two special requirements:

1. One serving should come from a citrus fruit or other source of vitamin C daily.

2. At least every other day one serving should come from a dark green or deep yellow colored vegetable to help fulfill the vitamin A requirement.

Two other servings of any vegetables and fruits, including potatoes, will round out this group.

Just because a person is on a calorie-restricted diet, he need not eliminate potatoes completely. Potatoes, especially when prepared whole including the skin, provide small quantities of important nutrients. The more surface area exposed in preparation—that is, the smaller the potatoes are cut up or sliced—the fewer the nutrients. The potato's most significant supply of nutrients lies just under the skin. Sweet potatoes supply significant quantities of vitamin A, plus additional iron. Generally, it is what we put on the potatoes—butter, sour cream—that makes the calories mount. Eaten plain and whole, the potato can be a worthwhile diet component.

Where are you on the Vegetable Continuum? Write your initials where you are now. Write your name where you would like to be.

Vegetable Continuum I

How much do you eat?

```
VEGETARIAN :   :   :   : XXXX   :   :   : : VEGETABLE
VIRGINIA   ──────────────────────────────   AVOIDER
                                             ABIGAIL
```

Open comment:

Vegetable Continuum II

How do you take your vegetables?

DISGUISE 'EM :____:____:____: XXXX :____:____:____ SWALLOW 'EM
   DENISE   WHOLE SALLY

Open comment:

BREAD-CEREALS GROUP

Selections of whole grain and enriched breads or cereals as well as rice and enriched macaroni, noodles, and spaghetti round out the daily diet recommended in the Four Food Groups. Flour enriched with thiamin, riboflavin, niacin, and iron substantially contributes to the fulfillment of the suggested requirements for these nutrients. Whole grain breads and cereals utilize the entire kernel, including the nutrient packed germ as well as the bran. Bran (along with dried fruits, nuts, seeds) is an excellent source of dietary fiber, an essential component for good health.

Perhaps one of the most palatable and psychologically rewarding of foods is homemade bread. The sight, smell, and texture makes the twenty-minute kneading process an enjoyable activity. Yeast breads are especially intriguing. Mixing flour, yeast, salt, and water can result in the most flavorful Italian bread. These simple breads are surprisingly low in calories—but have several people on hand to help you eat the bread when it comes out of the oven. Even a strong-willed person has trouble resisting seconds or thirds of hot, homemade bread.

Following the suggestions of the Four Food Groups Guide will supply the average, healthy American with nearly all of the nutrients considered necessary for growth and health. Despite criticism by leading nutritionists, who are concerned that the classification is confusing and that it doesn't provide adequately for iron, the Four Food Groups provide an excellent foundation for prudent and pragmatic nutrition.

For the adult, the simple 2-2-4-4 combination can be easily remembered: two servings from the meat group and two from the milk group; 4 servings from the bread and cereal group and 4 from the fruit and vegetable group (remembering to get a rich serving of vitamin C daily and a dark-green or yellow vegetable every other day).

Rank order the Four Food Groups, assigning your favorite number one, and your least favorite number four. Then list several of your favorite foods in each group.

___MILK GROUP	___MEAT GROUP
___VEGETABLE-FRUIT GROUP	___BREAD-CEREAL GROUP

FOOD KNOWLEDGE VS. FOOD EXPERIENCE

Knowledge alone will not change behavior. Many people *know* much better than they *do*. Cigarette-smoking doctors and overweight nutritionists are just a few examples. Ultimately, it is your values, not your knowledge, which guide your life through time and space. But we need knowledge to inform our values.

Occasionally we find ourselves in situations where we feel motivated to combine knowledge with action.

For example, I *know* about liver. I know that nutritionally it is a fantastic food. Nevertheless I had not consumed liver for well over twenty years. The reason: I don't like it! Recently, however, I ordered an Italian dish in a restaurant and, much to my dismay, I found the spaghetti mixed with chicken livers! Here I found myself in a situation gently nudging me to alter my food habits bringing them in line with my food knowledge. I decided to consume the liver (mixed heavily with tomato sauce, which I hoped would disguise the taste) and much to my surprise, found it reasonably palatable.

My knowledge of the nutritional qualities of liver had not been enough. If I had not been placed in a situation gently urging me to experiment with this food alternative, I doubt if I would ever have altered my experience. People change, however, and it is wise to continually reevaluate former choices and possibly change in ways that were not feasible previously in our lives. Generally, we are unwilling to risk—to deviate from learned patterns—when it comes to food alternatives. But taking a chance, when you are motivated and know it is worthwhile, can be an exhilarating experience.

Knowing vs. Doing

Answer the following questions as honestly as you can.

Record today's date at the top. Two weeks from now, reread your answers and note any changes.

_____
date

1. Has *knowledge* about the nutritional qualities of a particular food ever caused you to try it? Which food? Did it become part of your eating patterns?

2. Have you ever tried to avoid foods based on their lack of nutrition? Which ones? To what extent did you succeed?

3. How willing are you to *risk* new food alternatives? Do you try new foods that you never had before? Do you ever try again with a food you didn't like before?

4. Would you ever force yourself to consume nutritious foods? Is it easier for you to force yourself to avoid non-nutritious foods on a weight control program than it is to force yourself to eat nutritious foods?

PERSONAL DIET STUDY

One of the best ways to determine the nutritional adequacy of your diet is to do a long-range diet study. This involves a considerable amount of paper work, since you must record *all* the foods that go into your mouth. The following form has been provided for this purpose. It would be beneficial to do this Personal Diet Study periodically to keep a check on the nutritional adequacy of your diet. It's a lot of work but well worth it for the insight you will get into your actual nutritional patterns.

On the left side of the form list all the foods you have

DAILY FOOD INTAKE

_____
date

FOODS CONSUMED	APPROX. AMOUNT CONSUMED	CALORIES
BREAKFAST		
LUNCH		
DINNER		
SNACKS		

consumed during the day (breakfast, lunch, dinner, and snacks); how much of each you have eaten; and how many calories each food amounted to. Be sure to include *everything* you have taken in, however insignificant—mustard, catsup,

CHECKLIST

verdict

FOUR FOOD GROUPS ANALYSIS		
	CHECK PER SERVING	TOTAL CALORIES FOR EACH FOOD GROUP
MILK GROUP		
MEAT GROUP		
VEGETABLE-FRUIT GROUP One check for each fruit or vegetable		
"C" for each Vitamin C source		
"A" for each Vitamin A source		
BREAD-CEREAL GROUP		
EMPTY CALORIES		
MISCELLANEOUS		

onions, sugar, butter, jelly, chewing gum, etc. The goal is to be as complete and as accurate as possible. It's a good idea to have a good diet scale on which to weigh food. So often a dieter fails to accurately guesstimate the size of each serving. A diet scale takes the guesswork out of dieting.

The right side of the form is a simplified Four Food Groups checklist. For each food item that you consume, you should check some column on the Food Group checklist side of the form. Even junk foods like candy, and miscellaneous foods like coffee should be noted and checked. If you eat more or less than one suggested serving, record the appropriate fraction consumed. For example, four ounces of milk = ½ a serving.

For the Vegetable and Fruit Group, give yourself a check for *every* one of these foods you eat. Then, if the food is a source of vitamin C (such as citrus fruits, tomatoes, strawberries), also place a C within the subdivision of the Vegetable and Fruit Group. Similarly, dark green and deep yellow colored vegetables (such as string or wax beans, spinach, corn, kale, peas) which are rich in vitamin A, should be noted by an A within the subdivision. But remember: *all* fruits and vegetables—including those marked as rich sources of vitamin A and vitamin C—should be checked in the top part of the Vegetable and Fruit box.

If you have fulfilled your Four Food Group requirements for the day, draw a smile on the face on the top right hand side of the form. If not, draw a frown. If you're not sure, reread the chapter.

Do not change your normal eating patterns while you are carrying on the study. For this period only, try not to modify your diet to comply with the Four Food Groups. If you do, you may defeat the purpose of studying your nutritional pattern. Your goal is to find out what you normally eat.

Keep a checklist for the next five days. Run a similar check at least four times a year. Be honest.

REFERENCES

1. "Highlights from the Ten-State Nutrition Survey," *Nutrition Today*, July-August, 1972, pp. 4-11.

2. Lamb, Lawrence E., "Iron and Anemia," *The Health Letter*, 4, 1974: 4.

3. Paige, David M., et al., "Lactose Malabsorption and Milk Rejection in Negro Children," *The Johns Hopkins Medical Journal*, vol. 129, no. 3 (September, 1971), pp. 163-169; David M. Paige et al., "Lactose Intolerance in Peruvian Children: Effect of age and early Nutrition," *The American Journal of Clinical Nutrition*, 25 (March, 1972): 297-301; David Paige et al., "Response of lactose-intolerant children to different lactose levels," *The American Journal of Clinical Nutrition*, 25 (May, 1972): 467-469; Vinodini Reddy and Jitender Fershad, "Lactase deficiency in Indians," *The American Journal of Clinical Nutrition*, 25 (January, 1972), 114-119.

4. Lappe, Frances Moore, *Diet for a Small Planet*, New York: Ballantine Books, Inc., 1971.

The Role of Activity in Weight Control

I am convinced that inactivity is the most important factor explaining the frequency of 'creeping overweight' in our modern Western societies.[1]

JEAN MAYER

According to English law, life does not begin until "quickening" occurs. Quickening is the first recognizable movement of the fetus in the uterus, and it generally occurs around the fourth or fifth month of pregnancy. From quickening until death, movement is a sign of life; it is basic to our existence.

Man alive is man in motion. Death is the complete cessation of activity. A body at rest tends to stay at rest. The less we move, the less we desire to move. Eventually, we develop patterns of inactivity that, once established, are extremely difficult to change. The majority of people today are hypokinetic—we don't move enough. We ride rather than walk, sit rather than stand, and lie down rather than sit. This love of ease can lead to "dis-ease."

Reflect on the long-range consequences of inactivity patterns as you complete the following values exercise.

A Caution to Everybody

Consider the auk:
Becoming extinct
Because he forgot to fly,
And could only walk.
Consider man,
Who forgot how to walk
And learned how to fly
Before he thought.[2]

OGDEN NASH

1. What is your reaction to this poem?

2. React to Robert M. Hutchins' statement: "Whenever I feel like exercise, I lie down until the feeling goes away."

3. Does your own personal philosophy lean more toward regular activity or inactivity? Give several reasons for your point of view, whichever it may be.

INFLAMMATORY DISEASES

The majority of overweight people in the American society are victims of two insidious inflammatory diseases: sedentary-itis and spectator-itis.

Sedentary-itis is an inflammation of the muscles we sit on.

It is characterized by the motto: "Why expend energy when you don't have to?"

It appears that we have lost our founding forefathers' appreciation of hard work and enjoyment of the sweat of effort. We look for the easiest way to do things. No one really knows what caused this activity freeze, but surely television, automation, and the many laborsaving devices of a highly technological society have contributed to our love of ease.

Where did we go wrong? When we were children, our parents were always asking each other, "Where do the kids get all their energy?" Children have boundless amounts of energy *because* they are energetic. It snowballs. Energy that is expended is not wasted. It's invested in ourselves and pays immediate dividends by increasing our capacity to be active. Look at a group of children in a playground. Notice anything? Usually the most active kids are also the ones who are of normal or slightly below normal weight.

Somehow, though, the child learns to slow down his activity patterns. One reason this occurs is that a child is placed in a system that restricts his movements and discourages his desire to move. Movement.may be restricted if adequate recreation opportunities are not provided for children. Restricting a child's movement runs counter to his biological need and can result in frustration. After awhile that frustration will seek an escape hatch. If the escape hatch chosen is not socially acceptable, the child may be punished for his misbehavior with further restriction of his movements— "You must stay in your room"; "You can't go out and play after dinner"; etc. And so the vicious cycle of inactivity begins. A child cannot, on his own, find constructive ways to realize his need for large motor expression; therefore, opportunities should be made available to children by their parents and teachers.

Too often, the structure and controls that are built into the school environment snuff the child's movement. Healthy physiological expression is often sacrificed by the educator in favor of developing intellectual expression. Even when the school does provide opportunities in physical education classes or during recess, teachers tend to restrict and control free movement "for the good of the group." When the active child who has been restricted to a desk all morning seeks to express himself through large motor activity, the teacher labels him as "wild" or "hyperactive."

Sometimes exercises or calisthenics are used as a form of punishment. Over time, exercise may develop negative associations and create within the child a dislike for any activity.

Spectator-itis, the second insidious disease, is an inflammation of the eyes due to overexposure to the television set or to the activities of athletes in a large sports arena. It is invariably accompanied by sedentary-itis. We who desperately need exercise sit there consuming high-calorie, low-nutrient items such as soft drinks, beer, pretzels, potato chips, and hotdogs, watching physically-fit persons maintain their level of fitness. It just doesn't make sense!

Effortless Excesses

List the man-made mechanical and electrical devices (e.g., electric can opener) you most frequently use that save you steps, limit your energy expenditure, or create a state of activity freeze.

1. _____

2. _____

3. _____

4. _____

5. _____

6. _____

7. _____

8. _____

9. _____

10. _____

Mark your devices with the following codes:

E = those utilizing electricity
G = those utilizing gasoline or other fuel
$ = those requiring an initial outlay of twenty-five
     dollars or more
@ = those used while you are sitting down
* = your three favorites
K = those found in the kitchen
W = those associated with your work, including
     housework
X = those you could most easily do without for a year
     or more
O = the two you would find most difficult to give up
     for one year

1. What, if anything, does this strategy reveal to you
   about your use or abuse of laborsaving devices?

2. Has advertising persuaded you to buy products that may really be unnecessary?

BATTLING THE LAW OF INERTIA

Our highly mechanized and automated society places such a high value on saving steps, that movement has come to seem almost unnatural. Have you ever gone for a walk and been offered a ride by friends driving past? When you graciously refused their offer, did they become insulted, or look at you as if you were crazy because you'd rather walk?

If you hope to become and remain active, you may have to plan ahead for the activities that you enjoy. You can schedule the more vigorous activities for days when you exceed your caloric allowance.

As activity becomes a regular part of your normal daily routine, it becomes less awkward. But the first step is the hardest. Our habitual desire to remain inactive may make it necessary to do something radical to break the inactivity pattern.

A basic law of physics suggests that a body at rest tends to stay at rest. The human body at rest has an additional restraint—it's called a brain. Thanks to our higher level of consciousness, we can think up ingenious rationalizations and excuses for why our own particular body should stay at rest. We must constantly wage war against this indolent intelligence if we ever hope to enjoy the many benefits of the active life. Below are a number of motivational quotes that may help you overcome the inertia of your body at rest.

If you're not using your body, you're not using your head.

Don't dig an early grave with your knife and fork.

Exercise builds your life, not just your body.

You can't push a button for good health, but you *can* push yourself away from the table.

Give yourself a gift; add better years to your life by adding more life to your years.

It's rarely too late to start, but it's usually too soon to quit.

It's not a matter of what you *can* or cannot do, but of what you *want* to do.

THE DOUBLE BIND OF INACTIVITY

Most dieters try to lose weight only by cutting their caloric intake. Unfortunately, the body may interpret a diminution of calories as a famine, and react by slowing down the metabolism. Conversely, when your activity level increases, the body reacts by increasing the metabolic rate, figuring that food must be just around the corner. This increased metabolic rate is maintained for about twenty-four hours. Therefore, the active person is burning up more calories even while asleep than his friend who has restricted his food intake but is as sedentary as ever.

Paradoxically, inactivity can increase the appetite. There appears to be a regulatory center in the hypothalamus gland called the appestat which balances caloric intake and expenditure. This appestat becomes functional only when an individual remains moderately active. The appestat is not sensitive enough to deal with extremes. If too little activity is engaged in, the balance it maintains is lost.

The overweight individual requires more calories to do the same task as an individual of normal weight. It's as if you were carrying a weight strapped around your waist. Your system is overloaded by excess poundage and you require more energy to do the same amount of work. This may be the major reason for the cyclic nature of inactivity and overweight.

As a person becomes less active, which usually happens after you finish school, the appestat is thrown out of kilter. You eat slightly more and begin to gain weight because of inactivity and excessive eating. This combination puts weight on faster than either factor would working singly. As the individual's weight increases, it takes greater effort to engage in even simple movements. As the difficulty of exerting effort increases, activity levels decrease, and the appestat remains jammed. Now the person is overeating more than ever.

Eventually, the individual tends to become stabilized at the overweight, inactive level. Stabilization occurs when calories used balance out the number of calories consumed. Because he is carrying an extra load, the overweight person needs to consume an enormous number of calories to give him enough energy to maintain his restricted activity.

This ball and chain effect keeps the individual inactive because his overweight condition makes even minimal effort fatiguing. You can verify this by deliberately overloading your own system the next time you take a walk. Fill your pockets with rocks or carry a small child. After several minutes of walking you will begin to get the point. But don't stop there. Be sure to walk up a flight of stairs to get the full effect of carrying excessive weight. You will see what the overweight individual experiences with every movement he makes. The only exception is in the swimming pool. Fat makes you buoyant, so the more overweight a person is, the fewer calories he needs to keep himself afloat!

EXERCISE VS. ACTIVITY
VS. MOVEMENT

The word exercise often connotes a physical education class in which a group of people do jumping-jacks, sit-ups, and push-ups to the cadence set by the drill instructor. That is one form of movement, but few of us would choose calisthenics as the activity we most enjoy. I prefer the term activity, which conjures up fewer negative associations. Activity, in turn, is based on movement. The more we move the more active we are. And to be physically fit, we must be very active indeed.

Many people who claim they are active actually move very little. "How do you get your activity?" "Oh, I play tennis." Yet, if you observe the average person on the court, you will probably notice that he only swings if the ball is hit right to him. He rarely moves his feet, and consequently is hardly active at all. Calories consumed in playing a set of tennis can vary tremendously, depending upon how much and how vigorously the person moves. The "hit-it-right-to-me" player might better be designated as playing *at* tennis.

Activities

Below, make a list of your favorite activities.

Indicate next to each activity how much you engage in it daily or weekly.

Star the ones that involve a considerable amount of movement—the way *you* participate.

Place a double star next to those activities that involve a great deal of movement utilizing the large leg muscles.

1. _____

2. _____

3. _____

4. _____

5. _____

Movement is more than just a periodic workout. Movement should become a pattern of life. We need to assess the degree to which we move and figure out ways to move more if we hope to increase our caloric expenditure.

Many of my colleagues consider themselves quite active physically. They work out in the gymnasium for 30 minutes almost every day. However, let us put this half-hour of activity into the total context of their normal life patterns.

Each one drives to work, parking as close to the building as possible. He takes the elevator up to his office and sits at a desk and works. His work includes activities such as writing, dictating, opening books, reading, using a finger to dial the telephone, standing up, pulling open a drawer in the file cabinet, and sitting back down again. Occasionally, he may stand up and take a walk to the nearest bathroom. On the way back, he may pilfer a piece of candy from someone else's desk. During lunchtime he and some friends take the elevator down, hop into their cars, drive to the gymnasium, play basketball vigorously for thirty minutes, shower, dress, go back to the car, up the elevator, and back into the office for another four-hour shift of sedentary-itis. The rest of the day's activities consist of driving home, sitting down with the daily newspaper, opening the mail, walking to the table to eat dinner, and, following dinner, relaxing in front of the television set, exhausted from the day's "activities."

With the exception of the half-hour game of basketball, this constitutes the normal activity pattern for most Americans. Because of the basketball game, my colleague erroneously believes that he has gotten sufficient exercise for the day. He thinks he is active and physically fit, when in actuality, he has only been active for approximately thirty minutes out of the total day.

It would be more beneficial to establish a pattern of life in which there is activity throughout the day. A person who walks to work, walks up and down steps, goes out for an evening walk, and tries to be generally active rather than sedentary during most of his day may actually be better off than someone who exercises strenuously for a fixed period every day. Walking is one of the most underrated activities. We would all do ourselves and our society enormous benefit if we recovered our leg-power.

Sports vs. Walking[3]

But the faithful exercisers are a very small minority. And even their dedication to a favorite form of muscle-flexing tends to dwindle with each passing birthday. In their forties, perhaps even before, they falter. Going to the gym is for most a dreary ritual, and exercising at home is even drearier. The demands of business, career, family, edge the pleasures of sports into an ever narrower corner. Tennis and skiing are seasonal, and each year it seems more of a drag to get into condition again.

Golf is also seasonal in much of the country. The golfers generally stay with the game, but long before their legs give out they are riding rather than walking over the course, because it takes less time or is just so seductively easy. And there is always the expense in time and money, to say nothing of the effort of getting to the scene of the sport, which for city dwellers is considerable.

Walking has none of these disadvantages. Anybody who is not disabled can walk, whatever his age or the state of his muscles. Its playing field is as near as the street at one's front door; it requires no equipment, no lessons with a pro, no expenditure beyond the price of an extra pair of shoes per year, if that. Walking is the cheapest exercise in time, money, and energy. It is the most accessible and most generally available. Simple as it is, it is listed as a "best" exercise by the physical fitness experts and recommended as a health preserver and, for some of their patients, an outright life saver by the doctors.*

1.   What sports or exercises have you participated in?

2.   Are these feasible activities to continue for the rest of your life? Please comment on each activity.

---

* *The Magic of Walking* by Aaron Sussman and Ruth Goode. © 1967 by Aaron Sussman and Ruth Goode. Reprinted by permission of Simon & Schuster Inc.

3. How much walking do you do daily?

4. Would you consider making walking your activity?
   Make a list of the places that you could walk to as a
   means of transportation, and as a recreational
   activity.

Activity, Adolescents and Adipose Tissue[4]

*Instead of merely counting the calories a fat girl
consumes, obesity experts are now translating her
daily activity into calories—that is, finding how
much energy she uses up in a day, and how this
balances with the energy she takes in as food
(which is also measured in calories). By observing
fat girls swimming, playing volleyball, taking gym,
they have learned that these girls remain remarka-
bly motionless. In the swimming pool they are
likely to do a dead man's float while others are
practicing their crawl. Lack of activity explains why
a girl who doesn't eat excessively can still become
fat. If two teen-agers of the same weight eat equal
amounts of food, the one who takes a half-hour's
brisk walk daily will be in the neighborhood of
fifteen pounds lighter at the end of a year.*

*During the teen years boys typically slim down
while girls gain more fat. The probable explanation
is that boys are increasing their physical activity
while girls are decreasing theirs almost to the
vanishing point. Gym periods, often held only
twice a week, give a girl a bare ten minutes of actual*

exercise, and many, pleading menstrual discomfort, manage to skip gym frequently. The experts believe that differences in exercise habits explain why city girls are plumper than those from rural areas and why Massachusetts girls weigh more than those from sunny California.

1. Do you feel that your excess poundage is due to excessive calorie intake, lack of appropriate, regular activity, or a combination of both?

2. When you engage in various activities, are you an active or passive participant? How do you know?

3. Do you generally get out of breath after brief activity?

4. Do you mind sweating?

5. List several commonsense ways of increasing your activity patterns.

MOVEMENT VALUE

The amount of energy, or calories, we expend each day depends on the kinds of activity we engage in. The following chart will help you assess the total number of Movement Value points you score in a day. Each activity has been assigned a movement value in relation to all other activities. Multiply the points listed for a given activity by the amount of time you spend in that activity during a 24-hour period. If you have engaged in any activities that are not listed, estimate their appropriate movement value in relation to the others given.

Note your total Movement Value hours for the day _____ .

Estimate the approximate points by which you could realistically increase your total Movement Value if you consciously make a concerted effort to do so _____ .

Note the date you plan to start increasing your total Movement Value score _____ .

The higher the Movement Values in your life, the more calories you are burning up through voluntary muscular activity. Compute your daily Movement Value score for about a week every month. If it decreases, it's time for you to do something about your way of life.

MAJOR MISUNDERSTANDINGS ABOUT ACTIVITY

1. "To affect your weight, the activity must be concentrated." It *is* true that to lose one pound of body fat—3500 calories—a person would need to chop wood for seven hours, play volleyball for eleven hours, walk thirty-five miles, or climb the Washington Monument fifteen times!

DAILY MOVEMENT VALUE SCORE

Activity	Relative Movement Value	Hours Per Day	MV X Time
Sleeping, lying down	0		
Sitting, reading, watching TV, socializing	1		
Light activity: standing, driving, dressing	2		
Light housework: dusting, bed making, cooking	3		
Walking: strolling at 2.5 mph	4		
Light industrial work: painting, carpentry	5		
Walking: striding at 4 mph	6		
Moderate recreation: dancing, canoeing, ping pong, golf, volleyball, cycling 6 mph	7		
Heavy work: masonry, digging, haying, pick and shovel, cycling 10 mph	8		
Heavy recreation: jogging, walking up steps or hills, running, mountain climbing, tennis, skiing, handball, cycling 13 mph	10		
TOTAL		24	

Based on this, people rationalize that if it requires so much effort to lose one pound of body fat then it is not very realistic to include activity in their weight control plan. Using the same logic, however, calorie restriction would not make sense either, since an enormous amount of food would have to be eliminated in order to lose one pound of body fat.

We know, of course, that this is not true—the effects of calorie restriction are *cumulative*. Well, so are the effects of activity. It is not necessary to do all the activities in one continuous bout, any more than it would be to try to lose a pound a day through dieting. A man could chop wood for thirty minutes a day, and in fourteen days he would lose one pound of body *fat* (not water from sweat). A person could walk one mile per day, and in approximately one month lose one pound of body fat, provided his eating habits and other activities remained unchanged. This realistic but moderate change in physical activity would result in a twelve-pound weight-loss per year!

Consider the cumulative effects of the following, seemingly insignificant, change in activity patterns: A stenographer, sixty-three inches tall and weighing 120 pounds, uses 87.7 calories per hour operating a mechanical typewriter. She changes to an electric typewriter and her energy expenditure falls to 72.9 calories per hour. Each hour 14.8 calories are saved, which for a six-hour day amounts to almost ninety calories; in a five-day week, it adds up to 445 calories. If her food intake and other physical activity remain unchanged, she will gain one pound of body weight in about eight weeks, just because she had changed to an electric typewriter.[5]

2. "An increase in activity also means an increase in appetite." Since many people eat out of sheer boredom, it would almost be more true to say that a decrease in activity means an increase in appetite. Actually, it is the balance between what is taken in and what is expended that is most crucial to weight control. After several hours of vigorous activity the appetite of the sedentary individual might actually increase.

Too inactive a life appears to throw the normal balancing of eating versus activity out of kilter. Research has demonstrated that when a sedentary individual engages in a half hour or more of vigorous physical activity, his appestat becomes more accurate in regulating his food intake.[6]

Jean Mayer, a renowned Harvard University researcher, notes that rats exercised between one and two hours a day actually consume slightly fewer calories than unexercised rats. Rats exercised two or more hours did eat more, but this did not result in weight gain. The increased activity balanced out the increased caloric intake. During periods of extremely low activity levels, food intake actually increased and so did body weight. When rats were exercised to exhaustion—more than five hours of activity—both food intake and body weight decreased.[7]

Appestat Continuum

Are you satisfied with the current balance between your calorie intake and your energy output? Would you like to embark on a program to gradually increase your level of activity?

Write in your initials to indicate where, at this point in your life, you fall on this continuum. Write your name where you would like to be on this continuum.

Give some reasons for your desire to change your position, along with ways you plan to change your behavior.

Appestat Continuum

INDOLENT :   :   :   :   **XXXX**   :   :   :   :   ENERGY-
IKE ————————————————————————————————— EXHAUSTING
ERNIE

Open comment:

BREAKING THE CYCLE OF ACTIVITY RESTRICTION

Most of us are locked into a cycle of activity restriction. Our philosophy of doing things the easy way is so deeply ingrained into our lives that we may not even be aware of its pervasive influence. *(See top of page 163.)*

If you make a conscious effort, this cycle of activity restriction can be interrupted. Friends, books, personal determination, values reassessment—any or all of these may motivate you to begin an activity program. After about six weeks of increased activity you'll actually begin to experience a rejuvenation of physical and psychic energy! You will have developed endurance and increased your tolerance to the buildup of lactic acid, an end product of metabolism that can cause the feeling of fatigue. Further motivation to maintain the increased activity levels will come from your friends, who will make encouraging comments about the changes they have observed.

Cycle of Activity Restriction

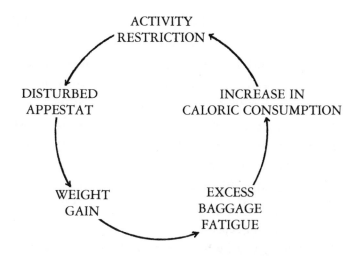

However, this revitalization can only begin if you take the first step—that giant step toward renewed vim and vigor.

Cycle of Regular Activity

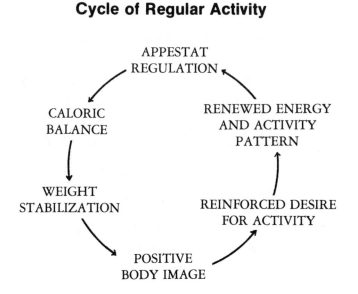

THE BEST ACTIVITIES
FOR LOSING WEIGHT

The most efficient weight-loss activities are those that use the large leg muscles. An ancient proverb states, "I have two doctors—my left leg and my right." Generally, any activity that involves walking, running, climbing, or jumping is good.

Walking briskly (striding, not just strolling) is one of the simplest and best exercises available to almost everyone. No special equipment is needed, nor do you have to rely on anyone else to make up a team. It's the most natural exercise of all.

Walking also has psychological benefits which in turn result in physical benefits for the dieter. We all know that when we are depressed, anxious, tense, we tend to do a lot more snacking than when we're feeling good. Walking works off tension and reduces the urge to feed ourselves to make ourselves feel better.

Walking: An Antidote to Tension[8]

Tension is probably the most widespread complaint that people bring to their physicians. It gives them headaches, backaches, elevated blood pressure. It keeps them awake at night or tossing in unrestful sleep. It makes them inefficient at work and irritable at home. They take expensive pills and go on expensive vacations to get rid of their tension. The pills and the vacations work, to a degree, about as well as the dieting for overweight. They win relief for a while, but the tension is always there, stealing back into muscles and nerves and tying body and mind into little knots.

Walking is the direct physiological answer to tension. Even a short brisk walk can drain away anger and anxiety, solve a problem, untangle the knots both physical and psychological. Walking as a regular part of the day or week draws off tensions before they turn into headaches and insomnia that need pills, or backaches that take expensive orthopedic skills to relieve them.

*Most people do not know that walking, commonplace ordinary walking, can perform these wonders for them. Or if they have been told, they do not believe it. Yet it is a relatively simple interaction of body and mind, psychosomatic and somatopsychic, which does not require a course in physiology to understand. The mechanisms by which walking restores and preserves muscular, nervous, and emotional health are a heritage as ancient as the first man.**

1. What techniques do you currently use to relieve tension?

2. Have they consistently worked?

3. Have you ever tried walking as a tension antidote?

4. Would you consider *regular* walking if you believed it could serve as a preventive factor against tension, irritability, and insomnia?

5. Do you believe a regular program of walking can do the things suggested above?

* *The Magic of Walking* © by Aaron Sussman and Ruth Goode. Reprinted by permission of Simon & Schuster, Inc.

6.   What plan would you be ready to undertake with regard to walking?

SPOT REDUCTION

Many people wish to reduce specific areas of their bodies without necessarily affecting the remaining areas. Isolated fat reduction is almost impossible to accomplish.

Adipose tissue is deposited throughout the body in a pattern that is common to most people. Although each individual has his own distinctive patterns, the following order of fat deposition generally applies: hips, buttocks, thighs, waist, chest, upper arms, lower legs, face, and fingers.

To the disappointment of most dieters, weight also comes off in a predetermined manner, which is generally the reverse order from the way it went on: fingers, face, upper torso, chest, waist, and lastly, thighs, rear, and hips.

Many women ask: "How can I reduce in all areas of my body except my breasts?" Unfortunately, there is no answer; breast shrinkage is often one of the first noticeable results of a weight-loss program.

For the most part, doing trunk exercises will not reduce excessive fat deposits around the trunk. Walking will not burn up fat in the thigh area. The fat burned up by physical activity is drawn from stored up deposits throughout the body; some of it even comes from the deeper tissues rather than from the tissues immediately under the skin.

LOSING INCHES BUT NOT POUNDS

Activity programs that isolate specific groups of muscles may not effect a weight loss, but can be of great benefit, especially for relatively inactive individuals. Even though your scale may show no change, you will profit both physiologically and psychologically from this kind of activity. Relatively inactive muscles groups will eventually deteriorate and lose their tone. Eventually they will feel and look flabby.

Muscles respond to increased activity by increasing not only in strength but also in tone and weight. The toned muscle holds larger quantities of blood protein. As the muscle tones up, the flabbiness of the muscle is lost and you may lose inches around the muscle without losing any weight. This is due to the increased denseness of the toned muscle fiber, which contains much more fluid than a flabby muscle. If you are interested only in weight loss, this could be discouraging. However, losing inches instead of pounds is as important to your health and appearance as weight reduction. You will feel trimmer. Your clothes will hang differently and you will notice that inches have been lost, and that your muscles feel tighter. People will start to comment that you've lost weight—even though you know better. So don't become discouraged because the scale is not cooperating; eventually, it will.

One important group of muscles is the abdominals, which in Americans are notoriously weak. The pot belly needn't, but too often does, characterize middle age. We tend to avoid movements that would strengthen these muscles. Walking and running don't do much for the abdominal muscles. Sitting for long periods of time further weakens this muscle group. Up until recently, sit-ups have been thought to strengthen the abdominal muscles. Recent findings, however, suggest that sit-ups are only minimally effective in strengthening the abdominal muscles; most of the effort of a sit-up strengthens the hip flexor muscles in the back, rather than the abdomen.

However, there is a way of performing sit-ups so as to

benefit the abdominal muscles. Instead of lying with your legs stretched out, bend your legs at the knee, either by keeping your feet close to your buttocks, or by placing your calves on a chair or bench. Now do your sit-ups from this position. People who may perform well with straight-leg sit-ups find that their performance of bent-leg sit-ups is markedly reduced—often by more than half.

The strengthening and toning of the abdominal muscles will not cause you to lose significant stores of fat around the abdominal area. Fat loss results from a calorie deficit. What you will notice is a reduction in your waist size. Many individuals claim a waist reduction of two or more inches within a month or less just from doing sit-ups with their legs bent.

BENEFITS OF A PROGRAM OF ACTIVITY

The rewards of breaking out of the passivity and inertia that characterize most Americans can be great. As hard as it may be to start and stick to a regular program of activity, once having determined upon it, it will be easier and easier to continue in it as the physical, psychological and social gains become noticeable. When you feel better in body and mind, when people begin to respond to you more positively, you will find that you are so full of energy and good will that you will actively enjoy your new life style.

My Personal Benefits from Activity

In the chart provided below, keep a running written record of every benefit you have derived from a more active life.

List the date you began each activity, and the date you first noticed each benefit.

Activity	Date Begun	Date Benefit Noticed	Benefit

Overfed—Undersexed

Is it possible that overfed people have shifted their major erogenous zone to their mouths? Freud might call these people orally fixated, i.e., their erogenous zone never dropped down to their genitals.

The hypothalamus gland regulates two appetites—the appestat, which regulates one's desire or hunger for food, and the "hornistat"—which regulates one's desire or hunger for sex. Could it be that in fat people there is a mix-up in the transmission of messages to the hypothalamus?

Herein lies a problem. Do overweight persons overfeed

* Courtesy of the Milk Foundation, Chicago.

themselves as a cover-up for their sexual hang-ups? Perhaps the grossly overweight individual unconsciously knows that his excess weight makes him sexually undesirable to his partner, thereby reducing his need to perform sexually.

1. Do you agree with the ideas expressed above?

2. If your partner were to become over-fat, do you think that your physical responsiveness to him or her would be different? Explain.

3. How is your sex drive affected by your weight?

4. Do you think a change in your weight would produce a change in your sex life?

5. It has been said that American men are very poor lovers because they suffer from "too-itis" disease— too tobaccoed, too fat, too physically unfit, too anxious, too laxy, and too alcoholed. What's your opinion?

FROM MOVEMENT TO FITNESS

Would you like to be able to go through a normal day's routines without undue fatigue, and still have energy left in reserve with which to meet emergency situations? Then you are interested in physical fitness. Physical fitness comes from movement, but not just any old kind. Movement with a purpose enables you to utilize larger quantities of oxygen in a given period of time, which results in greater biological efficiency.

You may have broken out of your cycle of movement restriction. You may even have developed a movement orientation to life. But most likely you are still not physically fit. The achievement of physical fitness requires a concentrated effort to fully utilize every movement to derive from it its maximum potential.

PRINCIPLES OF PHYSICAL FITNESS

The following principles should help you convert your activity program into an effective physical fitness program.

1. Enjoyment.   If you do not enjoy an activity, by all means don't engage in it! Enjoyment serves as a strong motivator to maintain your movement orientation to life. If jogging or even walking is not your bag right now, simply select an activity that you do enjoy. People change; in the future you may become interested in an activity that you now reject. Variety is the spice of life and a change of activities may play an important part in bolstering your motivation to overcome hypokinesis.

    In choosing activities you enjoy, try to remember that it is particularly helpful to engage in those using the large leg muscles. Look specifically for activities that do not rely on special equipment or on other people. Sometimes the purchase and maintenance of special equipment becomes prohibitive, and the difficulty of making arrangements with partners may discourage you from continuing the activity.

2.   Regularity.   To be of value, the activity must become a regular part of your life. It is recommended that you engage in an activity a minimum of three times per week on non-consecutive days. Don't be a "weekend athlete." Dr. Warren Guild of Harvard Medical School warns, "Anyone who exercises only on weekends is asking for trouble."[9] Perhaps you can pattern your activity schedule after the work week—five consecutive days for activity, two for "relaxing." However you do it, the important thing is to establish your activity as part of your normal routine. The choice of schedule is yours. What's important is making a choice, and consistently following through with it. Once you've reached the level of fitness you desire, two or three non-consecutive days per week is all you need to maintain that level.

3.   Overload.   In this context, overload may be defined as engaging in an activity beyond the point of comfort. If you feel comfortable walking a mile in twenty minutes (that is, at three miles per hour), then *that* activity pace will not improve your fitness level; it will only maintain the level you are at now. To improve your fitness level, the activity must be severe enough to demand more from the system than it can perform comfortably. You should be moderately fatigued upon finishing a given activity. As a rule of thumb, in activities involving the cardiovascular system, you should be out of breath for one full minute upon completion. Remember, you can take your time in reach-

ing this level. Do it gradually; resist the temptation to persist in an activity way beyond your physical limits in the hope that fitness will be achieved more rapidly.

4.   Progression.   To consistently improve your fitness level, you must progress beyond the point at which your system has adjusted to the overload. When a given activity no longer causes you to be out of breath for a full minute, or does not leave your muscles feeling "worked out," your body has adjusted to that level of activity. At that point, you will have to overload again if you desire further improvement in fitness. To increase your fitness level would require:

a)   increasing the *duration* of the activity. For example, increase your running-walking distance to 2 miles, then to 2-1/2 miles, etc.

b)   increasing the *speed* at which you engage in the activity. For example, if walking one mile in 20 minutes (3 miles an hour) no longer causes you to be out of breath, then decrease the total time to 15 minutes (four miles an hour). This increase in speed should cause you to be out of breath. As your system adjusts to this walking speed, perhaps you can then decrease the time to 12 minutes for a mile if you desire further improvements in your level of fitness.

c)   combining both approaches—increasing duration and speed. For example, instead of doing one mile in 20 minutes, increase the distance you travel to 1-1/4 miles, and at the same time increase your speed to 3-1/4 miles an hour. This way you should finish your workout (1-1/4 miles) in a little over 20 minutes.

THE BEST ACTIVITIES FOR FITNESS

According to Dr. Kenneth Cooper, author of *Aerobics*[10], the best physical activities are:

1. Running
2. Swimming
3. Cycling
4. Walking or striding, especially uphill
5. Stationary running
6. Handball
7. Basketball
8. Squash

These activities are listed in descending order of their ability to elevate your heart rate to its peak performance. Isometrics, weightlifting, and calisthenics do not even make his list of recommended activities because they do not sufficiently activate the organs that utilize oxygen.

One Woman's Liberation—From Fat, Fatigue, and Apathy[11]

> *I come from a family that suffers from a disease common to 50,000,000 Americans: overweight. (Incredible as it seems, 25 percent of this country's population is at least 15 pounds overweight.) My sister used to tip the scales at over 200 and my grandmother died weighing close to 300 pounds. I never had a weight problem while I was growing up because I was active—I played girls' basketball*

and in college I took the required physical education courses—but like many others my family certainly didn't encourage regular exercise as a way of life. . . . After a regular program of exercises, I became two sizes smaller. I weighed less. My eating habits were automatically controlled. I was less tense, more energetic and slept better. My resting heart rate decreased from 82 to 57 beats per minute. My self-image was definitely enhanced. I was aware of my husband's pride in me.*

1. Of the benefits attributed to a regular exercise program according to the above article, rank order the three that would be most important to *you*:

    — losing inches   — improved self image
    — losing weight   — less tension
    — eating less   — more energy
      without trying   — sleeping better
    — heart functions   — gaining approval
      better

2. Mildred Cooper claims that, thanks to exercise, "I can enjoy the luxury of eating what I please without worrying about calories." Does this statement convince you to start and persist in a regular physical fitness program?

* from: *Aerobics for Women* by Mildred Cooper and Kenneth Cooper © by Mildred Cooper & Kenneth Cooper. Reprinted by permission of the publisher, M. Evans & Co., Inc. New York, N. Y.

3. Mildred Cooper and her husband like to exercise by running. At this point, what activity would be *your* choice as the foundation of your exercise program?

4. Would you choose jogging as your fitness activity? Why, or why not?

CHOOSING A FITNESS PROGRAM

As we have indicated, the program you select should be enjoyable and varied and should escalate in its degree of severity. When you begin, moderate activities should be the rule. But once you have developed a sound foundation, you should progress to more taxing activities. The most successful program is one that remains flexible and adaptable to the actual and changing tastes and interests of its follower.

Listed below are sources which will supply you with prepared programs. Your choice will depend upon your needs, interests, and fitness level. The important thing is that you *choose* one. Discuss it with your doctor and, if he approves, get going on it. Too many people just *talk* physical fitness; they exercise their mouths more than their muscles. In fitness, actions speak louder than words. As an old Chinese proverb has it:

> What I hear, I forget.
> What I see, I remember.
> What I do, I know.

GENERAL SOURCES:

1. H. P. Hood and Sons in support of the President's Council on Youth Fitness, *Family Physical Fitness, Tests and Plans.*
2. Fred W. Kasch and John L. Boyer, *Adult Fitness: Principles and Practices,* National Press Books, 1968.
3. G. Mann and H. L. Garrett, *Over 30: An Exercise Program for Adults.* Nashville: Aurora Publishers, Inc., 1970.
4. *Metropolitan Life's Exercise Guide for Men and Women,* Metropolitan Life Insurance Company, 1968.
5. Robert R. Spackman, Jr., *Exercise in the Office,* Southern Illinois University Press, 1968.
6. A. Sussman and R. Goode, *The Magic of Walking,* New York: Simon and Schuster, 1967.

MATERIALS AVAILABLE FROM PRESIDENT'S COUNCIL ON PHYSICAL FITNESS AND SPORTS

To obtain these materials, write to: Superintendent of Documents, United States Government Printing Office, Washington, D.C. 20402

1. *Cureton's Basic Principles of Physical Fitness,* (1973-727-983/1184 3-1).
2. Thomas K. Cureton, M. D., *Trends of Research on Prevention of Psychological Aging and the Values of Exercise for Fitness and Health* (1973-727-932/779 3-1).
3. *Jogging Guidelines* (1973-727-986/789 3-1).
4. Stan LeProtti, *The Motivation Factor* (1973-727-984/787 3-1).
5. Jackie Sorensen, *Aerobic Dancing—a Rhythmic Sport,* (1973-727-933/780 3-1).

6. *Vigor: A Complete Exercise Plan for Boys 12 to 18,* (0-717-485).

7. *Vim: A Complete Exercise Plan for Girls 12 to 18,* (0-717-484).

NATIONAL PROGRAMS:

1. American Youth Hostels, Inc., 20 West 17th St., New York, N. Y. 10011

2. Appalachian Trail Conference, 1718 "N" St., N. W., Washington, D.C. 20036

3. *Bicycle Clubs Directory,* available from: Bicycle Institute of America, Inc., 122 East 42nd St., New York, N. Y. 10017

4. League of American Wheelmen, P.O. Box 3928, Torrance, California 90510

5. Sierra Club, 1050 Mills Tower, San Francisco, California 94104

LOCAL PROGRAMS:

1. YMCA's of the United States, 291 Broadway, New York, N. Y. 10017

2. State Councils on Physical Fitness

3. Bureaus of Recreation (state, city, and local)

4. Jewish Community Centers

FOR ADDITIONAL INFORMATION ON PHYSICAL FITNESS, WRITE TO:

1. American Alliance of Health, Physical Education Research, 1201 16th Street N.W., Washington, D. C. 20036

2. American Medical Association, 535 Dearborn St., Chicago, Ill. 60610

3. American Heart Association, 44 E. 22nd St., New York, N. Y. 10010

4. National Recreation and Park Association, 1700 Pennsylvania Ave. N.W., Washington, D. C. 20006

5. President's Council on Physical Fitness and Sports, 333 "C" Street S.W., Washington, D. C. 20201

IS IT WORTH THE PAIN?

Exercise has often been described as something unnecessarily painful. Some people consider exercise a form of masochism, or even torture.

No doubt you have, in your lifetime, experienced many painful situations other than exercise. In rank order, write the five most excruciatingly painful experiences you can remember.

Most Painful Experiences:

1. _____

2. _____

3. _____

4. _____

5. _____

Now list in rank order the most painful exercises you have done.

Most Painful Exercises:

1. _____

2. _____

3. _____

4. _____

5. _____

Star any painful experiences and exercises that resulted in something worthwhile.

Put X beside those experiences or exercises that you could do without.

How do you feel about pain being a necessary part of life?

Could you endure the temporary unpleasantness of eating liver or drinking milk, if you knew the benefits would be longlasting? Comment.

The Pace: Pain vs. Pleasure[12]

Only man enjoys what may harm him and avoids what may be good for him. Only wondering, seeking, clever man invents shortcuts to save work and deprives himself of the activity that can keep him healthy. Only man goes to excesses of ease and comfort that may do him harm.

People take to walking to avoid pain—the pain of illness or of the fear of illness—only when their physicians persuade them that the danger is real and present. But they will walk if once they discover that walking gives them pleasure—the pleasure of well-being, of better looks, of peace of mind, the pleasure of new and refreshing experience for their senses and their emotions.

In our world, walking has suffered from a bad press. Recent waves of physical fitness mania have equated walking with fifty-mile hikes, which are painful in the extreme for most people even to think about. Many men take into later life an association of walking with the dreary marches of their military training. Many women complain that walking tires them, when in fact, they do not walk at all. They go window-shopping, stopping and starting, standing and looking. This is an enjoyable occupation but it has no resemblance to the tireless swing of rhythmic walking . . .

. . . And not nature walking alone, but city walking or any other walking must be a direct experience. Until you have walked, the magic of walking will remain something of a mystery. Until

you have known the rhythm of a good walk in your own muscles, the movement of air on your own face, the changing scenes with your own eyes, you do not know what you have been missing.

But if once you have felt the refreshment of mind and body that is the reward of a good walk, then you are on the way to making walking a pleasure that will go with you through the rest of your life.*

1. Describe an occasion in which you experienced *pain* from walking. Did that experience turn you off to walking?

2. What is your current attitude about walking? Comment as to your pain/pleasure concept of walking.

3. When was the last time that you went for a rhythmic, non-stop stride for over:

one mile   _____   _____
                 date   *your feelings*

two miles   _____   _____
                 date   *your feelings*

three miles _____   _____
                 date   *your feelings*

---

* *The Magic of Walking* by Aaron Sussman and Ruth Goode. ©1967 by Aaron Sussman and Ruth Goode. Reprinted by permission of Simon & Schuster, Inc.

four miles ——————————   ——————————————
                       date   *your feelings*

five miles ——————————   ——————————————
                       date   *your feelings*

4. How often do you go for a good, rhythmic walk?

WHAT ACTIVITY WILL NOT DO

Activity will probably not decrease your life-span. However, because studies are incomplete as yet, we cannot promise that activity will increase your life-span either.

Activity will not necessarily prevent infections. Even though it may help strengthen the body's lines of defense against infections, it has never been proven to prevent them.

Exercise will not make you muscle-bound. Some athletes purposely train themselves with weights to develop that rippling muscle effect that is highly prized in Mister America contests. The average participant in a physical fitness program will find that normal exercise increases muscle flexibility and elasticity, rather than the reverse.

Exercise will not cause a woman to take on more masculine characteristics. Physical structure is determined by heredity and hormonal levels. Physical fitness programs operate within the limits of heredity and hormones. Women concerned about developing unseemly muscles can be assured that their normal flow of estrogen helps produce an extra layer of fat just under the skin, which keeps muscles from protruding.

WHAT ACTIVITY WILL DO

If your activity program meets the criteria of enjoyment, regularity, overload, and progression, you will in due course experience most of the following benefits:

The confidence of knowing that you are actively engaged in taking the most prudent steps necessary to sustain your well-being. The satisfaction of feeling that you have taken the shaping of your life into your own hands.

A healthy release of emotional tensions and pressures. Activity functions as a safety valve, reducing stress and lowering the body's production of cholesterol.

A sense of relaxation, which will give you a more positive attitude toward your work.

A higher metabolic rate.

Increased strength and endurance of the heart. Every time your heart beats, a greater volume of blood is pumped through your system.

Heightened activity of the blood, increasing the oxygen-carrying capacity of the cardiovascular system.

Lowered pulse and blood pressure rates at work and at rest.

Lower lactic acid levels during inactivity and an increased tolerance for lactic acid during work and vigorous activities.

A better chance of avoiding severe heart disease. Among those who do suffer from heart disease, there is a higher mortality rate for inactive individuals than for those who are active. Even after a heart attack, should it occur, regular activity will reduce the possibility of recurring heart dysfunctions.

Delayed onset of arteriosclerosis (a hardening of the arteries), and possibly prevention of cerebral-vascular accidents (strokes).

Easier childbirth and recovery.

Less frequent low back pain, which is often due to weak abdominal muscles.

Better digestion, absorption and utilization of food.

Less frequent constipation. Inactivity can cause lack of muscle tone in the small and large intestines and reduce peristaltic movement in the intestines.

Sounder sleep.

An improved capacity for relaxation.

Improved adjustment to acidemia, an excessive accumulation of acid in the blood.

Improved coordination.

Faster recovery rate from any strenuous work task.

Great assistance in losing weight, as regular activity:
    Balances the appestat;
    Increases the metabolic rate;
    Decreases the needed food intake compared with the formerly sedentary rate of consumption;
    Burns up substantial calories when calculated over long periods of time.

Better metabolism; the kidneys excrete metabolic acids more rapidly.

Steadier blood sugar levels.

Reduced rate of respiration. Once moderate physical fitness has been achieved, an individual breathes with less difficulty in performing a given exercise. Breathlessness is also delayed.

Reduced chance of blood clotting. Bedridden or severely inactive individuals run a high risk of developing clots. Drugs are often prescribed to "thin the blood" and reduce the possibility of clot formation.

Lower levels of uric acid, which may cause gout.

Write down any additional benefits of a fitness program that apply to you personally.

A Heart's Eye View of Overweight

Oh, my aching heart! Another pound of fat! That's another half mile of blood pathways I must pump the vital life substance through!

I am not getting any overtime pay. Nor do I get any rest! No wonder I'm so tired all day. Even if I belong to a person of normal weight, I work hard—I beat over 100,000 times per day, or nearly 40,000,000 times a year. I pump more than 4,000 quarts of blood daily through 8,000 miles of blood pathways. While the rest of the body sleeps, I do a work load equivalent to carrying a 30-pound pack to the top of the 102-story Empire State Building.

This excess weight is so discouraging, I think I'm going to

have to retire early. I even have difficulty "breathing" with all this adipose padding. My own artery has its tubes all clogged up.

Damn you, owner—have a heart!

1. This heart speaks of "retiring early" because of the excess baggage it is burdened with. At your present weight, how tempted is your heart to retire early?

2. What is your gut-level response to your heart's plea and threat?

3. List several alternatives that are available to you to help reduce your risk of heart disease.

4. Commit yourself in writing to doing at least two things at your earliest opportunity.

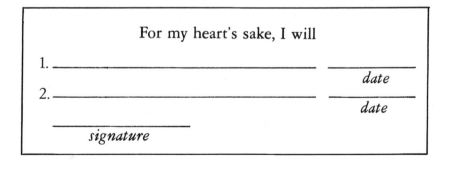

5. Verbally share with _____ at least one
    name

of your plans of action and ask for support in putting it into operation.

REFERENCES

1. Mayer, Jean, Exercise and Weight Control, *Postgraduate Medicine,* Vol. 25, 1959, p. 325.

2. Nash, Ogden, *Verses from 1929 On,* Boston: Little, Brown, & Co., 1959.

3. Sussman, A., & R. Goode, *The Magic of Walking,* New York: Simon & Schuster, 1967, p. 24.

4. Lake, Alice, "Obesity," *Seventeen Magazine,* Oct., 1969, p. 129.

5. Miller, B. F. and J. J. Burt, *Good Health,* (2nd edition), Philadelphia: W. B. Saunders, 1966, pp. 378-379.

6. Mayer, *loc. cit.*

7. Mayer, Jean, *Overweight: Causes, Cost, and Control,* Englewood Cliffs, N. J.: Prentice-Hall, 1968, p. 73.

8. Sussman & Goode, *loc. cit.* p.27.

9. Guild, Warren R., "Don't be *Just* a Weekend Athlete," *Today's Health,* July, 1966, p. 46.

10 Cooper, Kenneth, *Aerobics,* New York: Bantam Books, 1968, p. 15.

11. Cooper, Mildred & Kenneth, *Aerobics for Women,* New York: Bantam Books, 1972, pp. 11-16.

12. Sussman & Goode, *loc. cit.* pp.28-29.

Developing a
Calorie Consciousness

Calories do count. Your caloric figures probably explain the present condition of your figure. Even if you have a poor head for figures, calorie counting can become second nature to you. You will soon develop expertise in counting two kinds of calories—those you take in and those you expend.

You should become calorie conscious in order to give yourself greater freedom and flexibility in planning your own diet. Begin to commit to memory the caloric values of the foods you normally consume.

Calorie consciousness also involves becoming familiar with your personal caloric expenditure for the wide range of physical activities you perform. You should begin to calculate your caloric needs for each day, accounting for each moment of a twenty-four-hour period. Once you have analyzed your total caloric expenditure per day, you will have a much better idea of how many calories you can safely consume without gaining weight.

WHAT IS A CALORIE?

An ounce is a unit measure of weight. An inch is a measure of length. A calorie is a unit measure of heat. One calorie (sometimes referred to as a kilocalorie or k-calorie because it is larger than a calorie used in physics) is the amount of heat required to raise one kilogram of water one Centigrade degree.

A calorie does not measure weight; it's a measure of heat—potential heat. When speaking of body metabolism, the terms "heat," "energy," and "calories" can be used interchangeably. During the process of metabolism, the stored, potential energy in a calorie is burned up, thereby producing heat. Calories are accumulated through the food we ingest. Once deposited in the body's bank account, the calorie can be spent only through heat production. There are no magical withdrawals from this bank account without the heat produced through expenditure of energy.

A calorie is not an inch, nor is it an ounce. However, since a calorie has mass, it also has measurable weight. For example, 113 calories from a carbohydrate source weigh one ounce. Since fat is the most concentrated source of energy—two and a quarter times more concentrated than carbohydrates—255 calories from a fat source weigh one ounce.

Energy stored in the form of fat is nature's way of conserving space while preserving large quantities of energy. Obviously, a pound of body fat weighs the same as a pound of carbohydrate—16 ounces or 454 grams. The difference is in the caloric yield; the pound of fat theoretically yields 4,086 calories of heat energy and the pound of carbohydrate yields 1,816 calories of heat energy. Actually, 4,086 calories are not stored within a pound of body fat, for approximately 12% of the pound is accounted for by water retention; therefore, a pound of body fat yields about 3,500 calories.

WHAT IS WATER WEIGHT?

Water has weight but no calories. One pint of water (16 ounces) weighs one pound. Water constitutes the majority of body weight. Your body needs a certain amount of water to function. The body's conservation and utilization of its water supply is a very precise process. Interfering with this balance creates problems.

Weight gained through fluid retention is only temporary; your body wll eventually excrete the excess. Conversely, weight lost through excess water excretion, brought on by sweating or diuretics, is also temporary. Water balance must be maintained for physiological efficiency. A loss of water weight will show up quickly on a scale, but the body will quickly replace it once the imbalance has been felt.

Since water contains no calories it is not burned up. Water is released from the cell as a by-product of metabolism to help stabilize body temperature. The harder you work your body, the more heat it produces. Excessive heat production causes sweating, which in turn reduces the body temperature. Sweating eliminates water weight from the body, but no fat weight is lost. This principle is important to your calorie consciousness.

For example, if you were to drink 16 fluid ounces of water, your body would store no calories, but your weight would show a temporary increase of one scale pound. If you were to drink 16 ounces of cola containing sugar worth 210 calories, the same weight gain—one pound—would show up immediately on the scale. Over time the body will utilize the fluids from both sources to balance its water supply. However, the calories from the cola drink will remain part of your total weight, if not burned up. These 210 calories account for approximately 2 ounces of body weight in their carbohydrate form. If not used up by the system, these carbohydrate calories will be converted into fat calories weighing a little less than one ounce. About 16 unused pints of cola calories would result in approximately a one pound body weight gain!

Water balance is also influenced by salt and hormones. An excess of either of these two substances will cause the body to retain more fluids than it needs. This extra weight shows up on the scale, but when appropriate adjustments are made in salt intake, excessive fluid retention generally stops.

Just prior to menstruation, many women experience a bloated feeling, which is due to an increased production of the hormone progesterone. Just as salt retains water, progesterone retains fluid. After menstruation the water balance is reinstated. Women who are using the combination estrogen-progestin birth-control pill retain this fluid for the entire cycle. The sequential birth control pill (estrogen followed in sequence by progestin) appears to more closely simulate the normal cycle.

BEING SELECTIVE ABOUT CALORIES

If calorie counts are stored in your memory bank, perhaps they will be less likely to find their way into your body's calorie bank account.

If you consume 100 excess calories per day, you will gain about nine to twelve pounds per year. A daily excess of 50 calories would equal a 4 ½ pound weight gain per year.

If you want to avoid such disaster, you will have to become adept at calorie counting. When you are thoroughly familiar with the caloric values of various foods, especially foods within the same nutritional groups, you will find that you have much greater flexibility. Very soon you will reach the point where you can examine or plan a menu and choose portion controlled foods that are low in calories, nutritious—*and that you like.*

You will reach the point where you are automatically making mental computations of all the calories you are consuming as you go along. Instead of restricting you, keeping a running total in your head will actually give you greater freedom. If, at 10 AM, 4 PM, 7 PM, or 11 PM you are aware of how many calories you've had so far, and how many more you're still allowed, you will know whether you can have that extra cookie, glass of wine, piece of fruit. You will make choices that both please and satisfy you.

We all generally tend to overeat foods that are our favorites. It's a good idea to examine your favorite foods and the quantities in which you indulge in them and see if it is worth it. If you're limiting your caloric intake, the more you eat of one food the less room there is left for other foods. The choice is yours. Make it consciously and wisely.

Favorite Calorie Intakes

In the chart provided below, list your ten favorite foods, as well as the amounts you normally consume per serving. Using the Food Energy caloric values listed in the Food energy column in Appendix B, record the appropriate caloric content for the amount you consume.

Look over your list carefully. In view of what you now know about the nutritional value of various foods, are there any items on your list of favorites that you would now reconsider? Put a ? next to any such item.

Are there any items that you think are excessive? Put a — next to those foods that you think you should reduce in quantity. Which items are junk foods, providing mostly empty calories? Put J next to these.

Are there any items you would consider eliminating completely at this point? Mark these with an X.

Favorite Foods	Amount Per Serving	Calories
1.		
2.		
3.		
4.		
5.		
6.		
7.		
8.		
9.		
10.		

Choose the food that is your least favorite and figure out how many calories you would save in a month if you eliminated it completely. Multiply the calories per serving by how many times you would normally have eaten this food in a month.

CALORIE COUNTING

Calorie counting will eventually become automatic to you. At first it is a cumbersome procedure that requires memorization and much repetition for reinforcement. However, just as with memorizing the keys on the typewriter or piano, eventually the task becomes a skill, taken over by the autonomic nervous system. The following drill will help familiarize you with the caloric content of selected foods in different groups.

Playing the Calorie Game

In the chart below, the foods are listed in alphabetical order within each category. Your task is to place the foods in sequence according to their calorie content. Rank as number one the food you think is highest in calories in that group; then guesstimate the number of calories for that food. The correct answers are found at the end of this chapter.

Category	Food		Rank	Estimated Calories	Actual Calories
Drinks	Beer Cola Skim milk Whole milk	8 oz. 8 oz. 8 oz. 8 oz.			
Fruits-Vegetables	Apple Celery stalks Potato Potato chips	1 extra large 10 large 1 med. boiled 9 medium			
Snacks	Chocolate kisses Peanuts, salted Pizza, cheese Raisins	7 1 oz. ⅛ of 14″ pie 1 oz.			
Ice Cream	Chocolate Orange-ice Orange sherbert Strawberry Vanilla	1/6 qt. 1/6 qt. 1/6 qt. 1/6 qt. 1/6 qt.			
Soup	Chicken noodle Chicken w. rice Split pea Tomato	1 cup 1 cup 1 cup 1 cup			

Category	Food		Rank	Estimated Calories	Actual Calories
Fruits	Apple Banana Navel orange Peach Pear	1 medium 6 inch 1 large 4 oz. 1 medium			
Meat and Fish	Fish sticks, fried Hamburger on bun Frankfurter on roll	5 2 oz.			
Candy	Caramels Chocolate bar w. almonds Gum drops Jelly beans Marshmallows	3 1 oz. 20 10 4 large			
Juice	Grape juice Grapefruit juice, fresh Lime, fresh Orange juice Tomato juice	1 cup (8 oz.) 1 cup 1 1 cup 1 cup			
Alcoholic Beverages	Light ale, 4% proof Martini Scotch Ruby port	 8 oz. 2 oz. 1 ½ oz. 4 oz.			

100-CALORIE PORTIONS

To deal with calories in another way, it might be helpful to standardize the calorie content and vary the amount of food. The chart below will tell you what quantity of each food will supply 100 calories. This chart, based on tabulations by the U.S. Department of Agriculture, may be somewhat different from charts with which you are familiar. However, it makes comparisons easier and may help you realize the importance of controlling portions of certain foods.

100-CALORIE PORTIONS*

Food	Portion	Wt./Vol. (oz.)
Anchovies, canned	15 thin fillets	2
Apple, fresh	1 (3" diam.)	8
juice	¾ cup	6
pie	1/12 part (9" pie)	2
Applesauce	½ cup	4
Apricots, fresh	5 medium	6
canned	½ cup (2½ medium)	5
juice	⅔ cup	5
Artichoke	1 large	6
Asparagus, fresh	30 spears	20
canned	30 spears	24
Avocado	¼ fruit	1⅔
Bacon, broiled	2 slices	⅔
Bananas, fresh	1 medium	3½
Beans		
baked with pork	⅓ cup	3
lima, green, canned	¾ cup	5
string	3½ cups	14
Beef		
consomme	10 cups	80
corned	1 slice	1
loin (lean)	1 slice	1½
rib (lean)	1 slice	1⅓
roast	1 slice	2
sirloin steak (lean)	1 sm. slice	2
tongue	2 slices	1½

* Reprinted by permission of Pennwalt, Pharmaceutical Division, Rochester, New York

100-Calorie Portions (continued)

Food	Portion	Wt./Vol. (ounces)
Beer	½ can	6
Beets, fresh, cooked	4	8
Biscuit, baking pwdr.	one (2″ diam.)	1
Blackberries, fresh	40 berries	6
Blueberries, fresh	1 cup	5
pie	1/12 part (9″ pie)	1½
Bluefish, baked or broiled	1 piece	3
Bologna	2 thin slices	1⅔
Bourbon	1 jigger	1½
Bran, wheat	1 cup	2
Bread	1½ slice	1
Brie cheese	1 sm. wedge	1½
Broccoli	3 stalks	10
Brussels sprouts, cooked	1½ cups	7
Butter	2 sm. squares	½
Butterfish	1 piece	2
Buttermilk (whole)	1 cup	8
Cabbage, fresh, cooked	2½ cups	12
Cake		
angel	1 slice (2″)	1⅓
fruit	1 sm. slice	1
sponge	1 slice (2″)	1
Camembert cheese	1 wedge	1
Candy bar, chocolate	one piece	⅔
Cantaloupe	½ melon (5″ diam.)	15
Carrots, fresh, cooked	2 cups	10
Cauliflower, raw	3 cups	12
Celery, raw, diced	6 cups	18
Cheese		
American	small cube	1
cheddar	1″ cube	1
cottage	4 tbsp.	3⅔
sandwich, American	⅓ sand.	4
souffle	½ cup	2
Cherries, fresh	1 cup	6
Chicken, broiled	1 slice	2
roast	1 slice	2
Chocolate, sweet	sm. piece	⅔
Chow Mein	½ cup	4
Cider	¾ cup	6
Clams	6	5
Club sandwich	¼ sand	—
Codfish	1 slice	5

100-Calorie Portions *(continued)*

Food	Portion	Wt./Vol. (ounces)
Coffee, black	(no caloric value)	
Cookies, plain	1 medium (3″ diam.)	1
lady fingers	3	1
oatmeal raisin	1	1½
Corn		
canned	½ cup (creamed)	4
flakes	1¼ cup	1
Corned beef sandwich	⅓ sand.	—
Crabs, fresh	½ cup	4½
meat, canned	½ cup	4
Crackers		
cheese or oyster	20	1
normal size	3	1
saltines	7	1
Cranberries, fresh	1¾ cup	7
sauce	¼ cup	1½
Cream, heavy	2 tbsp.	—
Cream cheese	2 tbsp.	1
Cucumbers	3 whole (large)	24
Custard	1 cust'd cup	4
Custard pie	1/12 part (9″ pie)	2
Dates	4 dates	1
Doughnuts	½ d-nut	1
Duck	½ breast or 1 thigh	2¼
Eggs, raw	1⅓ eggs	2
whites only	7 whites	7½
yolk only	2 yolks	1
boiled	1⅓ eggs	2
Figs, fresh	3 small	4
dried	2 small	1¼
Flounder	1 slice	3
Frankfurter	1 sausage	1½
French dressing	1½ tbsp.	¾
Fruit salad	1 cup	8
Gefilte fish	½ cup	4
Goose	small slice	2
Grapefruit, fresh	½ fruit (4″ diam.)	8
juice, canned	1 cup	8
Grapes	1 lg. bunch (40)	5
Griddle cake	1 cake (4″ diam.)	2
Gumdrops	3 pieces	2
Haddock, cooked	⅔ fillet	5
Halibut	small piece	3
Ham, fresh, lean	slice	1

100-Calorie Portions (continued)

Food	Portion	Wt./Vol. (ounces)
Hamburger, lean	very sm. pat	2
Hash, corned beef	¼ cup	1½
Herring	⅓ herring	3
Honeydew melon	¾ (5″ melon)	10
Horseradish	20 tbsp.	10
Ice cream	⅓ cup	2
Ice cream soda	⅓ glass	2
Jam; Marmalade; Jellies	1½ tbsp.	1½
Kale	1½ cup	8
Kidney		
veal	1 kidney	3
beef	½ kidney	2⅔
Lamb		
chops	1 rib chop	2
leg or shoulder	1 sm. slice	2
Leeks	7 leeks	8
Lemon, fresh	3 lg. fruit	10
juice	1 lg. glass	8
pie	1/12 part (9″ pie)	1
Lentils, dried	2 tbsp.	1
Lettuce	2 heads	20
Liver, broiled	1 good slice	1½
Liverwurst	1 slice	1½
Lobster, fresh	⅔ cup	4
Luncheon meat	1 slice	1¼
Macaroni, elbow, cooked	½ cup	2½
Macaroons	2 (small)	1
Manhattan cocktail	½ glass	1½
Marshmallows	5	1
Mayonnaise	1 tbsp.	½
Milk		
skimmed	1¼ cup	10
whole	⅔ cup	5
non-fat solids	3½ tbsp.	—
Mince pie	1/16 part (9″ pie)	1
Mints		
cream	10 small	½
chocolate	1 large	¼
Muffins	1	2
Mushrooms, fresh	10	4
soup	½ cup	4
Mussels	8	4
Mustard	5 tbsp.	3
Mutton chops	½ chop	2

100-Calorie Portions (continued)

Food	Portion	Wt./Vol. (ounces)
Noodles		
uncooked	¼ cup	1
soup	1 cup	8
Oatmeal, cooked	¾ cup	5
Oil, cooking or salad	4/5 tbsp.	½
Okra	25 pieces	9
Olives, green	16 (ex. lg.)	—
ripe	12	—
Onions	2 medium (2½ ")	7
Onion soup	⅔ plate	6
Oranges, fresh	1 large	7
juice, fresh	1 cup	8
marmalade	1 tbsp.	1
Oysters	8-12 medium	5
Parsnips, raw	⅔ parsnip (large)	4
Pastrami	½ thin sl.	1
Peaches, fresh	2 medium	7
canned	2 lg. halves	4
Peanuts		
roasted	20	½
butter	1 tbsp.	½
Pears, fresh	1 large (3 " diam.)	6
canned	2½ halves	5
Peas, green, fresh	¾ cup	4
Peas, canned	¾ cup	3½
dried, split	2 tbsp.	1
soup	½ cup	4
Peppers, green	5	12
Pickles		
dill	6 large (1¾ x 4)	—
sweet	3 small (¾ x 2¾)	—
Pineapple, canned or fresh	2 slices	6
juice	¾ cup	6
Pizza (tomato & cheese pie)	3 " section (14 " pie)	1½
Plums, canned or fresh	4 fruits	6½
Pork		
chops, broiled	½ lean chop	2
Tenderloin, broiled	½ slice	2½
Potato		
boiled or baked	1 medium	3
mashed, white	½ cup	3½
chips	8 lg. pcs.	½
salad	¼ cup	2
soup	½ cup	4
Pretzels	2 large or 8 small	1

100-Calorie Portions (continued)

Food	Portion	Wt./Vol. (ounces)
Prune		
juice	½ cup	4
whip	½ cup	2½
dried or fresh	4 medium	1½
Puffed Wheat	2⅓ cups	—
Pumpkin pie	1/12 part (9″ pie)	2
Radishes	40 small	15
Raisins	2 tbsp.	1
Raspberries	1¼ cup	5
Red wine (dry)	1⅓ glass	4
Rhubarb, raw	6 cups	18
stewed	½ cup	4
pie	1/12 part (9″ pie)	1½
Rice, boiled	¾ cup	4
Rice Krispies	¾ cup	1
Roe: shad; salmon; cod	⅓ medium	2½
Rolls	1 medium	1¼
Roquefort, cheese	sm. wedge	1
dressing	1 tbsp.	1
Rye bread	1 slice	1½
Salami	⅔ slice	¾
Salmon		
fresh or canned	½ cup	2½
smoked	1-2 small slices	2
Sardines, canned	5	2
Sauerkraut	2½ cups	15
Scallops, raw	⅔ cup	4
Shad, baked or broiled	1 slice	2
Sherbets	½ cup	3½
Shrimp	15 medium	3
Syrup, maple or corn	1½ tbsp.	1
Soft drinks, carbonated	1 cup	8
Soy sauce	¾ cup	6
Spaghetti, cooked	¾ cup	4
Spinach, cooked	2 cups	12
Split pea soup	¾ cup	6
Squash		
summer, boiled	3 cups	21
winter, boiled	1⅓ cup	9
Strawberries, fresh, no sugar	2 cups	9
Sugar, cubes	4 lumps	—
powdered	2½ tbsp.	—
granular	6½ tsp.	—
Sweetbreads, calf	⅓	4

100-Calorie Portions (continued)

Food	Portion	Wt./Vol. (ounces)
Sweet potatoes	½ potato	2½
Swordfish	½ slice	2
Tangerines, fresh	2 large	7
juice	½ glass	4
Tomatoes, fresh	3	16
juice	2 cups	16
soup	1 cup	8
canned	2⅙ cups	—
Triscuit	5 wafers	1⅔
Trout	½ medium	3
Tuna fish, canned	¼ cup	2
Turkey	1 slice	2
Turnip, greens	2 cups	10
white	2½ cups	12
Veal		
breast	½ slice	2
steak	⅓	1½
cutlet	⅓	1½
Vegetable soup	1 cup	8
Waffles	1	1½
Walnuts	10 halves	½
Watercress	4 bunches	16
Watermelon	medium sl.	12
Wheat bread	1⅓ slices	1
Whitefish	⅓ portion	2
White wine (dry)	1½ glass	5
Yoghurt	⅔ cup	6

VARIATIONS WITHIN FOOD GROUPS

Variety is the spice of life; we do get tired of eating the same foods all the time. Often we shift from one food item to another within the same group assuming that the caloric value is more or less the same. This may not turn out to be so at all.

The following charts should familiarize you with the wide variations in calorie content that exist within groups of apparently similar foods. Differences come from the foods themselves, as well as from the form of preparation.

DIFFERENT CALORIC VALUES OF POTATOES
DEPENDING ON METHOD OF PREPARATION

(All values are for 100 gm, 3½ oz. servings)

TYPE OF PREPARATION	CALORIES
Raw White	76
Boiled, peeled	65
Boiled in skin	76
Baked, peeled after baking	93
Mashed, milk added	65-78
Mashed, milk and margarine added	94-120
French fried, frozen	220
French fried, fresh	274
Hashbrowns	229
Potato sticks	300
Potato chips, crisp	568

DIFFERENT CALORIC VALUES OF
VARIOUS FORMS OF MILK

(All values are for 8 oz. servings)

TYPE	CALORIES
Whole milk:	
3.5% Butter Fat Content	160
2% Butter Fat Content	137
1% Butter Fat Content	115
Skim milk	90-98
Butter milk	98
Chocolate-flavored milk	212
Half and Half	325
Egg Nog	474

DIFFERENT CALORIC VALUES OF BREADS
(All values are for 1 slice servings)

TYPE	CALORIES
Boston brown	100
Cracked wheat	65
French	63
Gluten	35
Italian	62
Profile	52
Protein	45
Pumpernickel	77
Raisin	62
Rye, light	53
Vienna	63
White	64
Whole wheat	57

DIFFERENT CALORIC VALUES OF COMMON SNACK FOODS

TYPE	APPROXIMATE MEASURE	CALORIES
Beverages:		
Carbonated, cola type	6 oz.	70
Malted milk	1 ½ cups	420
Chocolate milk (skim milk)	1 cup	190
Cocoa	1 cup	235
Vanilla ice cream soda	1 ½ cups	260

DIFFERENT CALORIC VALUES OF COMMON SNACK FOODS		
TYPE	**APPROXIMATE MEASURE**	**CALORIES**
Cake:		
Angel food	2" sector	110
Cupcake, chocolate, iced	1	185
Fruit cake	2 × 2 × 1½"	115
Cream puff, custard filling	1 average	245
Doughnut, plain	1 average	125
Doughnut, jelly	1 average	225
Doughnut, raised	1 average	120
Candy:		
Butterscotch	3 pieces	60
Candy bar, plain	1	295
Caramels	3 med.	120
Chocolate coated creams	2 average	130
Fudge	1 piece	115
Peanut brittle	1 oz.	125
Popcorn (with oil)	1 cup	65
Cheese:		
Camembert	1 oz.	85
Cheddar	1 oz.	105
Cream	1 oz.	105
Swiss (domestic)	1 oz.	105
Cookies:		
Brownie	2 × 2 × ¾"	140
Cookies, plain assorted	3"	120
Crackers:		
Cheese	5	85
Graham	2 med.	55
Saltines	4	70
Rye	2	45

DIFFERENT CALORIC VALUES OF COMMON SNACK FOODS		
TYPE	**APPROXIMATE MEASURE**	**CALORIES**
Nuts:		
Mixed, shelled	8-12	95
Peanut butter	1 tb.	95
Peanuts, shelled, roasted	1 cup	840
Pie:		
Apple	4″ sector	345
Cherry	4″ sector	355
Custard	4″ sector	280
Lemon meringue	4″ sector	305
Mince	4″ sector	365
Pumpkin	4″ sector	275
Sandwiches:		
Bacon, lettuce, tomato	1	280
Egg salad	1	280
Ham	1	280
Liverwurst	1	250
Peanut butter	1	330
Soups, commercial canned:		
Bean with pork	1 cup	170
Beef noodle	1 cup	70
Chicken noodle	1 cup	65
Cream (mushroom)	1 cup	135
Tomato	1 cup	90
Vegetable with beef broth	1 cup	80

DIFFERENT CALORIC VALUES OF COMMON SNACK FOODS		
TYPE	APPROXIMATE MEASURE	CALORIES
Miscellaneous:		
Hamburger and bun	1 average	330
Ice cream, vanilla	3 ½ oz.	130
Jams, jellies,		
marmalades, preserves	1 tb.	55
Potato chips	10	115
Sherbet	½ cup	120
Syrup, blended	¼ cup	240
Waffle	4 ½ × 5 ½ × ½"	210

HOW CALORIES ARE USED—ENERGY OUTPUT

As we said before, calories are stored up unit measures of heat. In order for this heat to be used, the body must burn the food through a process called metabolism. The body has three ways to burn calories.

1. *Basic Metabolic Rate (BMR)*. The basic metabolic rate is the number of calories used to carry on the basic life functions, such as circulation and respiration. The Basic Metabolic Rate differs for each individual. Generally, it is one calorie per kilogram of body weight per hour. To calculate the calorie cost of your Basal Metabolism:

    a. 2.2 pounds equals one kilogram. Divide your

weight in pounds by 2.2. This gives you your
weight in kilograms.

$$\underline{\hspace{3cm}} \div 2.2 = \underline{\hspace{3cm}}$$
your weight in lbs.   *your weight in kilos*

b. To compute your basal metabolism multiply your
weight in kilograms by 24. This is the amount of
calories used per day for your BMR.

$$\underline{\hspace{3cm}} \times 24 = \underline{\hspace{3cm}}$$
your weight in kilos   *your BMR*

2. *Specific Dynamic Action (SDA).* SDA is the amount
of energy required to digest and process the food you
consume. Carbohydrates, alcohol, fat, and protein all
require different amounts of energy to be processed.
Generally, SDA requires about 6% of total calories
consumed over a twenty-four-hour period. Calculate
your SDA by the following formula:

$$\underline{\hspace{4cm}} \times .06 = \underline{\hspace{2cm}}$$
total calories consumed daily   *SDA*

3. *Voluntary Muscular Activity (VMA).* VMA is the
number of calories you use for all your activities
beyond those necessary for life functions. VMA
varies considerably for each individual. VMA is the
caloric variable you have the most control over.

Certain drugs may slightly increase the BMR; high-protein diet may increase the SDA from six to eight or nine percent. But these alterations do not significantly affect total caloric expenditure. VMA, on the other hand, can be held down to a few hundred or boosted to a few thousand calories. If we remain relatively inactive, in a hospital bed, for example, VMA may account for only a few hundred calories a day. A lumberjack, whose occupation requires a large amount of muscular activity, can burn up as many as 2,500 to 3,500 calories in voluntary muscular activity over and above BMR. This person can eat like a horse and not show any signs of being fat because he also works like a horse. In fact, he may actually lose weight during the heavy work season because he cannot eat enough food to maintain energy equilibrium.

How much energy do you expend in twenty-four hours? The following chart should help you estimate your caloric output through Voluntary Muscular Activity.

Column one lists a usual day's activities.

In column two record in hours how much time you spend at the activity each day. Your time in hours should be calculated to the nearest quarter of an hour. When completed, this column should total twenty-four hours.

Column three lists a constant which represents the calorie rate expended per kilogram for each of the various activities. This constant is really an estimate which has been established by evaluating each activity in *relationship* to the other listed activities. Sleep does not actually have a negative caloric expenditure, but it does in relation to the other activities. If an

DAILY CALORIC OUTPUT THROUGH VOLUNTARY MUSCULAR ACTIVITY

Activity	Time Spent (to nearest ¼ hour)	Cal./ kg.	Cal./ kg./ Hr.
Dressing and undressing		.7	
Eating		.4	
Sitting		.4	
Dancing		3.8	
Walking		2.0	
Striding rapidly		3.4	
Driving a car		.9	
Writing		.4	
Reading		.4	
Mild exercise		4.5	
Severe exercise		8.0	
Sleep		-.1	
Other:			
TOTAL	24		

activity in which you engage is not listed, find a similar activity that is listed and estimate calories/kilogram.

The fourth column is derived by multiplying the duration of each activity by the calories per kilogram per hour.

Add up the figures in column four. Then multiply this figure by your weight in kilograms. This will give you the total number of calories you spend in Voluntary Muscular Activity over a twenty-four-hour period.

$$\overline{} \quad \times \quad \overline{} \quad = \quad \overline{}$$

$$\text{\textit{Total Cal./kg./Hr.}} \qquad \text{\textit{Wt. in kg.}} \qquad \text{\textit{Daily Calories for VMA}}$$

At best, this calculation is only an estimate of your total caloric output for a twenty-four-hour period. Be careful with your math, especially the decimal points and negative numbers. Careless errors might distort your efforts or render VMA useless. As a rule of thumb, the average American uses between 400-800 calories daily for VMA.

TOTAL CALORIC OUTPUT

To estimate your total caloric output for a twenty-four hour period, add up your BMR, SDA, and VMA.

BMR   _____

SDA   _____

VMA   _____

Total Calories Expended Daily   _____

As we compare and contrast our caloric output charts with our caloric input charts, we can better understand the hard facts of caloric balance. Consider yourself very active if your Voluntary Muscular Activity exceeds your Basic Metabolic Rate.

FOOD-ACTIVITY CALORIC EQUIVALENTS

Food contains calories. Activity uses calories. Excessive eating will take its toll unless something is done to counter it. *Quid pro quo* ("something in exchange for something") should become part of your unconscious caloric balancing act. "If I do such and such at the table, then I need to do so and so as an activity to balance it out." For every excess calorie you eat, there must be a counterbalancing activity period. If not, you will surely gain weight.

How long would it take to walk off a large apple? Run off a doughnut? Sleep off a chocolate layer cake? How long would it take to work off a glass of beer by walking? by golfing? by sitting? running? swimming?

The chart which follows will give you a relative idea of how many minutes it would take to work off various food items through various activities. For example, in fifteen minutes, you could walk off a boiled egg, bicycle off a glass of orange juice, or swim off a one-ounce caramel. The same caramel *could* be burned up even if you do nothing but sit around the house; however, it would take almost two hours!

ACTIVITY EQUIVALENTS

FOOD	QUANTITY	CALORIES	Sleeping	Reclining	Sitting and Writing / Standing or	Typing or Playing Piano	Driving a Car	Preparing Meals	Making Beds
CALORIES/ MINUTE			1.0	1.4	1.9	2.5	2.8	3.3	3.9
Apple	1 large	101	101	72	53	40	36	30	26
Bacon	2 strips	96	96	69	51	38	34	29	25
Banana	1 small	88	88	63	46	35	31	27	23
Beans, green	1 cup	27	27	19	14	11	10	8	7
Beer	1 glass	114	114	81	60	46	41	35	29
Bread and butter	1 slice, a pat	78	78	56	41	31	28	24	20
Cake	1 wedge	356	356	254	187	142	127	107	91

OF VARIOUS FOODS[1]

Ironing	Bowling	Golfing	Cycling 5.5 mph	Cycling 10 mph	Walking 3.5 mph	Striding 4.5 mph	Jogging	Playing Tennis	Playing Handball	Swimming	Walking up Stairs or Hills	Running
4.2	4.4	5.0	4.5	8.0	5.2	7.0	10.0	7.1	10.2	11.0	18.3	19.4
24	23	20	22	12	19	14	10	14	10	9	6	5
23	22	19	21	12	18	13	9	14	9	9	5	5
21	20	18	20	11	17	12	8	12	7	8	5	5
6	6	5	6	3	5	3	2	4	3	2	1	1
27	26	23	25	14	22	16	11	16	11	10	6	6
19	18	16	17	9	15	11	7	11	8	7	4	4
85	81	71	79	44	68	50	35	50	35	32	19	18

ACTIVITY EQUIVALENTS

FOOD	QUANTITY	CALORIES	Sleeping	Reclining	Sitting and Writing / Standing or	Typing or Playing Piano	Driving a Car	Preparing Meals	Making Beds
CALORIES/ MINUTE			1.0	1.4	1.9	2.5	2.8	3.3	3.9
Carbonated beverages (cola)	8 oz.	106	106	76	56	43	38	32	27
CANDY hard, all flavors	1 oz.	110	110	78	57	44	39	33	28
caramel	1 oz.	118	118	84	62	47	42	35	30
chocolate fudge	1¼"	118	118	84	62	47	42	35	30
Hershey bar	1-3/8 oz.	209	209	149	110	83	74	63	53
jelly beans	10	66	66	47	34	26	23	20	16
Carrot, raw	3 oz.	42	42	30	22	22	15	13	11
Cereal, dry	½ cup w/milk and sugar	200	200	143	103	105	71	61	51

OF VARIOUS FOODS

Ironing	Bowling	Golfing	Cycling 5.5 mph	Cycling 10 mph	Walking 3.5 mph	Striding 4.5 mph	Jogging	Playing Tennis	Playing Handball	Swimming	Walking up Stairs or Hills	Running
4.2	4.4	5.0	4.5	8.0	5.2	7.0	10.0	7.1	10.2	11.0	18.3	19.4
25	24	21	24	13	20	15	10	15	10	10	6	5
26	25	22	24	13	21	15	11	15	10	10	6	6
28	26	23	26	14	22	16	11	16	11	10	6	6
28	26	23	26	14	22	16	11	16	11	10	6	6
49	47	41	46	26	40	29	20	29	20	19	11	10
15	15	13	14	8	12	9	6	9	6	6	3	3
10	10	8	9	5	8	6	4	6	4	4	2	2
48	45	40	44	25	38	28	20	28	20	18	11	10

ACTIVITY EQUIVALENTS

FOOD	QUANTITY	CALORIES	Sleeping	Reclining	Sitting and Writing / Standing or	Typing or Playing Piano	Driving a Car	Preparing Meals	Making Beds
CALORIES/ MINUTE			1.0	1.4	1.9	2.5	2.8	3.3	3.9
Cheese, cottage	1 tbs.	27	27	19	14	11	10	9	7
Cheese, cheddar	1 oz.	111	111	79	58	44	40	34	28
Chicken, fried	½ breast	232	232	166	122	93	83	70	59
Chicken,	1 TV dinner	542	542	387	285	217	194	164	139
Cookie, plain	148/ lb.	15	15	11	8	6	5	5	4
Cookie, chocolate chip	1 average	51	51	36	27	20	18	15	13
Doughnut	1 average	151	151	108	79	60	54	46	39

OF VARIOUS FOODS

Ironing	Bowling	Golfing	Cycling 5.5 mph	Cycling 10 mph	Walking 3.5 mph	Striding 4.5 mph	Jogging	Playing Tennis	Playing Handball	Swimming	Walking up Stairs or Hills	Running
4.2	4.4	5.0	4.5	8.0	5.2	7.0	10.0	7.1	10.2	11.0	18.3	19.4
6	6	5	6	3	5	3	2	4	3	2	1.4	1.0
27	25	22	25	13	21	15	11	16	11	10	6	6
55	53	46	52	29	45	33	23	33	23	21	13	12
129	123	108	120	67	104	77	54	76	54	49	30	28
4	3	3	3	1	3	2	1	2	2	1	.8	.77
12	12	10	11	6	10	6	5	7	5	5	3	3
36	34	30	34	18	29	21	15	21	15	13	8	8

ACTIVITY EQUIVALENTS

FOOD	QUANTITY	CALORIES	Sleeping	Reclining	Standing or Sitting and Writing	Typing or Playing Piano	Driving a Car	Preparing Meals	Making Beds
CALORIES/ MINUTE			1.0	1.4	1.9	2.5	2.8	3.3	3.9
Egg, fried	1	110	110	79	58	44	39	33	28
Egg, boiled	1	77	77	55	41	31	28	23	20
French dressing	1 tbs.	59	59	42	31	24	21	18	15
Halibut steak	4 oz.	205	205	146	108	82	73	62	53
Ham	2 slices	167	167	119	88	67	60	51	43
Ice cream	1/6 qt.	193	193	138	102	77	69	58	49
Ice cream soda	1 glass	255	255	182	134	102	91	77	65

OF VARIOUS FOODS

Ironing	Bowling	Golfing	Cycling 5.5 mph	Cycling 10 mph	Walking 3.5 mph	Striding 4.5 mph	Jogging	Playing Tennis	Playing Handball	Swimming	Walking up Stairs or Hills	Running
4.2	4.4	5.0	4.5	8.0	5.2	7.0	10.0	7.1	10.2	11.0	18.3	19.4
26	25	22	24	13	21	15	11	15	11	10	6	6
18	18	15	17	9	15	11	7	11	8	7	4	4
14	13	12	13	7	11	8	7	8	5	5	3	3
49	47	41	46	25	39	29	20	29	20	19	11	11
40	38	33	37	20	32	23	16	24	16	15	9	9
46	44	39	43	24	37	27	19	27	19	18	11	10
61	58	51	57	31	49	36	25	36	25	23	14	13

ACTIVITY EQUIVALENTS

FOOD	QUANTITY	CALORIES	Sleeping	Reclining	Standing or Sitting and Writing	Typing or Playing Piano	Driving a Car	Preparing Meals	Making Beds
CALORIES/ MINUTE			1.0	1.4	1.9	2.5	2.8	3.3	3.9
Ice milk	1/6 qt.	144	144	103	76	58	51	44	37
Jello with cream	½ cup	117	117	84	62	47	42	35	30
Malted milkshake	12 oz.	502	502	359	264	201	179	152	129
Mayonnaise	1 tbs.	92	92	66	48	37	33	27	24
Milk	1 glass	166	166	119	87	66	59	50	43
Milk, skim	1 glass	81	81	58	43	32	29	25	21
Milkshake	12 oz.	421	421	301	222	168	150	128	108

OF VARIOUS FOODS

Ironing	Bowling	Golfing	Cycling 5.5 mph	Cycling 10 mph	Walking 3.5 mph	Striding 4.5 mph	Jogging	Playing Tennis	Playing Handball	Swimming	Walking up Stairs or Hills	Running
4.2	4.4	5.0	4.5	8.0	5.2	7.0	10.0	7.1	10.2	11.0	18.3	19.4
34	33	29	32	18	28	20	14	20	14	13	8	7
28	27	23	26	22	23	25	17	16	11	11	6	6
120	114	100	111	62	97	71	50	71	49	46	27	26
22	21	18	20	11	18	13	9	13	9	8	5	5
40	38	33	27	20	32	23	16	23	16	15	9	9
19	18	16	18	10	16	11	8	11	8	7	4	4
100	96	84	94	52	81	60	42	59	41	38	23	22

ACTIVITY EQUIVALENTS

FOOD	QUANTITY	CALORIES	Sleeping	Reclining	Standing or Sitting and Writing	Typing or Playing Piano	Driving a Car	Preparing Meals	Making Beds
CALORIES/ MINUTE			1.0	1.4	1.9	2.5	2.8	3.3	3.9
Orange	1 medium	68	68	49	36	27	24	21	17
Orange juice	8 oz.	120	120	86	63	48	43	36	31
Pancake, with syrup	1	124	124	89	65	50	44	38	32
Peach	1 medium	46	46	33	24	18	16	14	12
Peas, green	½ cup	56	56	40	29	22	20	17	14
Pie, apple	1/6 pie	377	377	269	198	151	135	114	97
Pie, raisin	1/6 pie	437	437	312	230	175	156	132	112

OF VARIOUS FOODS

Ironing	Bowling	Golfing	Cycling 5.5 mph	Cycling 10 mph	Walking 3.5 mph	Striding 4.5 mph	Jogging	Playing Tennis	Playing Handball	Swimming	Walking up Stairs or Hills	Running
4.2	4.4	5.0	4.5	8.0	5.2	7.0	10.0	7.1	10.2	11.0	18.3	19.4
16	15	14	15	8	13	9	6	10	7	6	4	4
29	27	24	27	15	23	17	12	17	12	11	7	6
30	28	25	28	15	24	17	12	17	12	11	7	6
11	10	9	10	5	9	6	4	6	5	4	3	2
13	13	11	12	7	11	8	5	8	5	5	3	3
90	86	75	84	47	73	53	37	53	37	34	21	19
104	99	87	97	54	84	62	43	62	43	40	24	23

ACTIVITY EQUIVALENTS

FOOD	QUANTITY	CALORIES	Sleeping	Reclining	Sitting and Writing / Standing or	Typing or Playing Piano	Driving a Car	Preparing Meals	Making Beds
CALORIES/ MINUTE			1.0	1.4	1.9	2.5	2.8	3.3	3.9
Pizza, cheese	1/8 pie	180	180	129	95	72	64	55	46
Pork chop, loin	1 chop	314	314	224	165	126	112	95	81
Potato chips	1 serving	108	108	77	57	43	39	33	28
SAND- WICHES club	1	590	590	421	311	236	211	179	151
hamburger	1	350	350	250	184	140	125	106	90
roast beef with gravy	1	430	430	307	226	172	154	130	110
tuna salad	1	278	278	199	146	111	99	84	71
Sherbet	1/6 qt.	177	177	126	93	71	63	54	45
Shrimp, French fried	3 oz.	180	180	129	95	72	64	55	46

OF VARIOUS FOODS

Ironing	Bowling	Golfing	Cycling 5.5 mph	Cycling 10 mph	Walking 3.5 mph	Striding 4.5 mph	Jogging	Playing Tennis	Playing Handball	Swimming	Walking up Stairs or Hills	Running
4.2	4.4	5.0	4.5	8.0	5.2	7.0	10.0	7.1	10.2	11.0	18.3	19.4
43	41	36	40	22	35	25	18	25	18	16	10	9
75	71	63	70	39	60	44	31	44	31	29	17	16
26	25	22	24	13	21	15	10	15	11	10	6	6
140	134	118	131	73	113	84	59	83	59	54	32	30
83	80	70	78	43	67	50	35	49	35	31	19	18
102	98	86	96	53	83	61	43	61	43	39	23	22
66	63	56	62	34	53	39	27	39	27	25	15	14
42	40	35	39	22	34	25	17	25	17	16	10	9
43	41	36	40	22	35	25	18	25	18	16	10	9

ACTIVITY EQUIVALENTS

FOOD	QUANTITY	CALORIES	Sleeping	Reclining	Sitting and Writing / Standing or	Typing or Playing Piano	Driving a Car	Preparing Meals	Making Beds
CALORIES/ MINUTE			1.0	1.4	1.9	2.5	2.8	3.3	3.9
Spaghetti	1 cup w/meat & to- mato sauce	396	396	283	208	158	141	120	102
Steak, T-bone, lean	3 oz.	235	235	168	124	94	84	71	60
Strawberry shortcake	5 oz. incl. berries & cream	400	400	286	211	160	143	121	103

Answers to Playing the Calorie Game *(page 195)*.

Drinks: 114, 105, 90, 160
Fruits-Vegetables: 133, 80, 76, 97
Snacks: 152, 162, 185, 80
Ice Cream: 200, 96, 177, 169, 193

OF VARIOUS FOODS

Ironing	Bowling	Golfing	Cycling 5.5 mph	Cycling 10 mph	Walking 3.5 mph	Striding 4.5 mph	Jogging	Playing Tennis	Playing Handball	Swimming	Walking up Stairs or Hills	Running
4.2	4.4	5.0	4.5	8.0	5.2	7.0	10.0	7.1	10.2	11.0	18.3	19.4
94	90	79	88	49	76	56	39	56	39	36	22	20
56	53	47	52	29	45	33	23	33	23	21	13	12
95	91	80	89	57	77	56	40	56	39	36	22	21

Soups: 60, 37, 145, 90
Fruits: 70, 85, 65, 35, 100
Meats: 200, 265, 245
Candy: 115, 150, 100, 105, 90
Fruit juice: 135, 95, 60, 110, 50
Alcoholic beverages: 100, 180, 110, 200

REFERENCES

[1] Adapted and expanded by Helen Derwin (student, Towson State College) from a chart in Frank Konishi's "Calorie Equivalents of Activity," *Journal of the American Dietetic Association*, March 1965, p. 187.

Konishi, Frank *Exercise Equivalents of Foods,* Carbondale, Ill.: Southern Illinois University Press, 1973.

Analysis of
Popular Diet Plans

Most popular diet plans work, but usually they fail to explain to the dieter why the plan works. Is this information omitted because the originators themselves have little regard for the principles of weight control? Or, perhaps they view the dieter as intellectually uninterested or unable to comprehend an intelligent explanation? Or maybe, just maybe, there is no sound basis for that particular plan. Often the plan's promoters submerge the explanation in pseudomedical jargon that few people could comprehend. The fact is that most "lose weight fastfastfast" diets succeed because of the nature of the dieter, not because of the diets.

WHY POPULAR DIETS WORK
(ON A SHORT-TERM BASIS)

Popular diets generally tell you what you want to hear: "Eat— or drink—all you want and lose ugly fat"; "Lose ten pounds in ten days"; "Break every rule in the book and still lose twelve pounds in the first week"; "Eat all you want and lose weight"; "Lose ugly fat while you eat the foods you love."

When they succeed, part of the success of the quick-weight-loss plans is due to the enthusiasm and zeal of the dieter. Under the spell of a new diet idea, you can, for a short period of time, happily avoid or restrict your intake of certain foods, such as carbohydrates. If a significant initial weight loss takes place, your devotion to the diet is temporarily strengthened, and you can extend your selective fasting for several more weeks.

Monotony is another factor that sometimes contributes to the success of the popular diet. Several popular plans claim that you can eat as much as you like, as long as you restrict your consumption to certain foods, such as high-protein items. Despite the carte blanche to gorge himself on unlimited quantities of high-protein foods, the dieter usually gets satiated with the regime and ends up limiting his intake voluntarily—just as the originators of the plan hoped he would. Provided he doesn't cheat by substituting other foods, he will lose weight because he has automatically reduced his total calories.

WHY POPULAR DIETS DON'T WORK (OVER LONG PERIODS OF TIME)

Failure to reeducate the dieter about why and how to sustain lifelong caloric restriction is one of the major faults of the quick-weight-loss plans. Dieters don't want to hear about the necessity for a lifelong program of reduced caloric intake and increased caloric usage through activity. So, in the formulation of quick-weight-loss diets, these principles are omitted.

Knowledge is extremely important in sustaining your motivation for a lifelong weight control plan. You can follow along blindly only just so long. Then your motivation will decrease if you can't see for yourself where you are headed. In almost any diet you may follow, you will inevitably reach a point where although your food intake decreases, your rate of weight loss slows down. At this point the need for knowledge is crucial. Perhaps this is why most fad diets fade out of our behavior after several weeks. To keep going beyond the initial burst of enthusiasm, and through the discouraging period where we seem to reach a plateau, we need faith in the soundness of the diet that only knowledge of its principles can supply. Deprived of this information, we give up, revert to our old eating habits with enthusiasm until we find a different quick-weight-loss plan to try. Thus the cyclic and dangerous yo-yo pattern of dieting is perpetuated.

Diets will work only as long as the individual limits total caloric intake. Consequently, to get fast results (without increasing caloric usage), many diet plans are unrealistically restrictive. They require too much self-discipline. Within a few weeks or months, the dieter has had enough. He goes back to his old eating patterns.

HARMFUL EFFECTS OF CRASH DIETS

High-protein, high-fat, low-carbohydrate diets have a high satiety value; that is, the meal stays with you longer, so, theoretically, you will eat less. But you pay a high price for your reduced appetite.

Conventional approved diets limit the total number of calories but maintain a balance between the various food groups in order to assure the body of its needed nutrients.

The person following a fad diet may be eating the same *number* of calories a day as a person following a more conventional recommended diet, but he loses weight faster because he is consuming the three basic foodstuffs—carbohydrate, fat, and protein—in different ratios. This change in foodstuff ratios causes weight reduction through water loss, which is not only temporary but also dangerous. The following chart contrasts the foodstuff ratios of a 2,000 calorie conventional diet and a 2,000 calorie low-carbohydrate diet.

Conventional Diet

Carbohydrate	50%-55%	= 1,000 calories
Fat	30%-35%	= 600-700 calories
Protein	15%-20%	= 300-400 calories

Fad Diet

Carbohydrate	10%-15%	= 200-300 calories
Fat	30%-40%	= 600-800 calories
Protein	50%-60%	= 1,000-1,200 calories

The person on the fad diet may experience a dramatic initial "weight loss," resulting from the drastic change in the percentages of carbohydrate, protein, and fat being consumed. But in return for this loss, he is suffering in other, less visible ways.

To function properly, the body needs blood sugar. The most convenient source of blood sugar is carbohydrates. When consumption of carbohydrates is severely restricted, the body gets its blood sugar from fat and protein sources or from the body's reserves. Fat in foodstuffs is about 30% water; protein between 50% and 70%. As fat and protein are used for energy, their waste products—fat yields ketones and water; protein yields uric acid and water—must be eliminated from the body. The water is eliminated; hence the rapid weight loss. But the body still must deal with the other waste products of this process, and herein lie the dangers of fad diets.

When significant quantities of protein are used for energy, the system is overloaded with uric acid. This acid combines with sodium to form sodium urate. The kidneys can only eliminate a limited amount of sodium urate. The uric acid not eliminated can produce gout and uric acid kidney stones, especially if the dieter does not drink at least two quarts of water daily. In extreme cases, a large back-up of uric acid can cause uremic poisoning or acidosis, and may even result in death.

Even the sodium urate that is excreted causes problems. With the excretion of sodium urate, salt is lost from the system. The loss of salt will also cause a further loss of water. Even if the dieter drinks a lot of fluids, severe salt loss can lead to dehydration. Dehydration, in turn, produces such symptoms as fatigue, fainting spells, mild nausea, headaches, and general irritability.

RATING THE DIETS

In an excellent exposé of fad and popular diets, Theodore Berland, in conjunction with Consumer Guide, rated all the popular diets. For the dieter who wants all of the facts, myths, and mysteries of popular weight control, this book is recommended.

The following list is reprinted with permission from *Consumer Guide Rating the Diets,* Publications International, Ltd., Skokie, Illinois, 1976. The diets are listed in order of safety and effectiveness, with the best and safest first.

The highest rating, four stars, is given the following diets which have a relatively large proportion of protein; no more than 30% of fat, with unsaturated fat predominant; and a minimum of carbohydrates (no less than 60 grams) and very little sugar:

New York City Dept. of Health Diet

Weight Watchers Diet

Diet Workshop Diet

Diet Watchers Diet

Diet Control Centers Diet

Prudent Diet (N.Y.: David White, 1973)

Redbook's Wise Woman's Diet

Antonetti's Computer Diet (N.Y.: Evans, 1973)

Dr. Glenn's Once-and-For-All Diet

But I Don't Eat that Much (N.Y.: Dutton, 1974)

Dr. Smith's Astronaut Diet

Bazaar's New 9-Day Wonder Diet

Planned Vegetarian Diets

The Wine Diet (N.Y.: Abelord-Schwinn, 1974)

The Yogurt Diet (Long Island City: Dannon)

Rated second best, three stars, because they pay little attention to the proportions of proteins, fats, and carbohydrates; or because they do not differentiate between saturated and unsaturated fats, are the following low-calorie diets:

Drug Companies' Substitution Diets
Ladies' Home Journal Family Diet
Ladies' Home Journal Computer Diet
Cadence Computerized Diet
Nutritional Diets
Amazing New You Diet
Mayo Clinic Exchange Diet
Easy, No-Risk Diet
Easy 24-Hour Diet
Overeaters Anonymous Diet
San Francisco Weight Loss Diet
(N.Y.: Arthur Fields, 1975)
Polly Bergen's Cheating Diet (N.Y.: Peter Wyden, 1974)

Also rated second best, three stars, because they pay little attention to the different kinds of fats, are the following low-carbohydrate diets:

Dr. Yudkin's Low Carbohydrate Diet (50 gr. carbohydrate)
American Diabetes Association (125-to-300 gr. carbohydrate)
Carbo-Cal (60 gr. carbohydrate)
Carbo-Calories (60 gr. carbohydrate)
Fat Destroyer Diet (various levels of carbohydrate)
N.Y. Times Natural Foods Low-Carbo Diet
(58 gr. carbohydrate)
Thinking Man's Diet (60 gr. carbohydrate)
Doctor Schiff's Diet (West Nyack: Parker, 1974)
Doctor's Metabolic Diet (N. Y.: Crown, 1975)

Rated two stars are the following high-protein diets:

Dr. Stillman's 14-Day Shape-Up Diet
Dr. Stillman's Quick Weight-Loss Diet
Fat Free Forever Diet
Gayelord Hauser's New Diet Does It
Petrie's Lazy Lady Diet
Petrie's Miracle Diet
Perlstein Diet
Weighing Game Organic Diet
Think and Grow Thin Diet

High-fat diets receive a low rating. *Consumer Guide* Magazine found only two usable because of their emphasis on low calories and on vegetable oils or unsaturated fats. These two were rated one star:

Dr. Arai's Eat and Become Slim Beauty Book
Dr. Fredericks' Low-Carbohydrate Diet

The following diets are not recommended because they do not fit either the criterion of longevity or that of safety to health:

Crenshaw's Lecithin-Vinegar-Kelp-B6 Diet
The Simeons Technique
Berman's Boston Police Diet
Van Fleet's Non-Glue Food Diet
Drinking Man's Diet
Banting Diet
Dr. Atkins' Diet Revolution
Atkins' Vogue Super Diet
Atkins' Cosmopolitan Dehungrificaion Diet
Dr. Taller's Calories Don't Count
Dr. Reinsh's Eat, Drink, and Get Thin Diet

Rice Diet
Dr. Stillman's Inches-Off Diet
Bananas-and-Milk Diet
Candy Diets
Grapefruit Diets
Ice Cream Diet
Zen Macrobiotic Diet
Zero-Calorie Diet (Fasting)

CRITERIA FOR EVALUATING WEIGHT CONTROL PLANS

Within the next few years, new plans based on "revolutionary discoveries" are sure to flood an already deluged market. In your own defense, you should be prepared to rate any diet plan that comes down the line. Of the following criteria the first three are the most important. The other criteria are not listed in order of importance, since their importance depends on the individual dieter's needs.

1. *WORKABILITY:* The plan you follow should be based on these principles of weight control: decrease caloric intake, increase caloric expenditure, or do both. If a plan suggests that you can eat unlimited amounts of foods in certain categories, you should question its *workability.* Eating calories in excess of your total caloric needs will eventually cause a weight gain, even on high-protein, high-satiety diets. The potential for gaining weight if you follow these high-protein diets over prolonged periods is real.

2. *NUTRITIONAL ADEQUACY:* If you are going to

be on a weight control plan for longer than a few days, you must seriously consider the nutritional adequacy of the diet. Your daily requirements of the fifty-plus essential nutrients should be met. A reducing program puts a strain on your body, so you must take special care to supply it with the needed nutrient materials. Therefore, we recommend that the diet you follow or develop for yourself be based on the Four Food Groups. The Four Food Groups will provide the average healthy American with nearly all the essential nutrients in approximately their proper amounts.

3. *SAFETY FACTORS:* In developing or selecting a personalized diet, you must be cognizant of certain safety factors and take the necessary precautions. The rainbow treatment of diet pills can kill. Restricting carbohydrate intake too severely may cause dehydration and significant loss of protein materials. You should even be cautious about taking vitamin pills while dieting. If you are following the Four Food Groups, you are getting all the essential nutrients, including vitamins.

4. *REEDUCATION:* A sound dietary plan will help reeducate you to sensible eating practices. Proper food selection, calorie contents of foods, energy balance, the role of activity, and the need for a lifelong surveillance of one's diet are some of the principles that the plan should mention. The goal of the plan should be to teach you what you need to know in order to direct your own weight loss program. Plans that are intended to be followed

slavishly and aim at creating a dependency are suspect. Even if they work, they may be doing more for their designers' pocketbooks than they are for your well-being. A plan which is selling good health should reeducate you so that you can direct yourself.

5. *BOREDOM AND MONOTONY:* If a diet is the same day after day it reduces one's motivation to follow it. Variety is the spice of dietary success. The plan should encourage you to unleash your creativity in selecting and preparing low-calorie foods.

6. *PALATABILITY:* A diet must taste good and fit into your social and cultural background. If, for example, you hate fish, many dietary plans, even nutritionally adequate ones, would not be right for you. Look for a diet that gives you many alternatives.

7. *COST OF THE PLAN:* Monetary considerations also play their part in realistic selection of a lifelong diet plan. How expensive are the special foods you will need to purchase? Is there a book that must be purchased as a guide? Are you being urged to join a diet club and pay membership dues? Does the diet push certain high-priced brand-name foods?

    Diet regulaton is a lucrative enterprise. Thousands of products and plans are available to members of our great overweight society. The annual ripoff of the American consumer through such schemes is estimated at about one billion dollars per year. Unless you prefer to surrender more money than you can realistically spare, it is recommended that you invest some time in finding a proper plan.

TAKING IT OFF TOGETHER:
THE GROUP APPROACH

Every individual is unique; your friends and neighbors are not necessarily like you. Yet your friends and neighbors are more like you than you suppose. Double-talk? Not really.

Each one of us has a different style of losing weight. You may benefit enormously from being lectured at. Your neighbor may find that his best motivation is knowing he must weigh in every Monday night. Someone else may stick to a rigid diet because he is paying membership dues. We are all motivated differently. But regardless of our differences, we all have similar needs. Within most of us is the need to belong, to be accepted, to be loved—for what we are, not for what others want us to be.

In *The Art of Loving,* Erich Fromm talks about the difference between "aloneness" and "separateness", and suggests that the answer to the problem of human separateness lies in love. However, if anyone in our society feels alone, separate, and *un*loved, it is the overweight individual. He is ostracized and set apart because of his corpulence.

Feeling desperately alone, many overweight people seek acceptance within and through a group. Membership in a diet club that cares can rebuild a person's self-confidence to the point where he can get himself together enough to restrict his caloric intake. The *esprit de corps* generated in some clubs is almost miraculous. You can feel the warmth and genuineness the moment you step inside the door.

Diet clubs have a great opportunity to capitalize on the group process. The group's singleness of purpose—to lose weight—promotes a spiritual enthusiasm that can motivate the members to adhere to even the most rigid plan. Every week they can have their motivational cups refilled. Praise, encouragement, and friendship are used as positive reinforcers. Personal problems are aired and shared. Together, the members are stronger than any individual is alone. There's a synergistic effect: one plus one equals more than two.

OVERCOMING THE CYCLE OF REJECTION BY JOINING CLUBS

Diet clubs accept people where they are at—fat. Overweight people, conditioned to society's rejection, are amazed and pleased with the club's acceptance of them as persons—not as fat people, but as individual, unique persons. As was indicated in the opening chapter, the individual working to become thin from within can be assisted by others in overcoming the cycle of rejection. Because of the diversity of its membership, a group can provide special psychotherapeutic value.

OTHER ADVANTAGES OF DIET CLUBS

Most clubs offer sound diet programs. At the outset they encourage or require medical clearance. Clubs rarely recommend crash programs. Their diets are usually well-balanced, safe, and realistic. Most clubs also have a maintenance plan to prevent yo-yo dieting. If you are the type of person who needs other people, then the group approach of taking it off together may be your thing.

DISADVANTAGES AND LIMITATIONS OF DIET CLUBS

In general, I am very much in favor of the group approach if that's your thing. I have seen clubs work fantastically well for hundreds of individuals. The following considerations, however, should be taken into account.

Joining a club can sometimes be costly. Certain clubs may charge a dieter up to $300 a year for membership.

Some profit-making clubs subtly encourage dieters to use the club's prepackaged, portion-controlled products, which may be effective, but may also be relatively expensive compared to your own prepared foodstuffs.

Many diet clubs distribute lists of recommended and of forbidden foods. Examine these lists carefully. Lists of forbidden foods may include food containing important nutrients, such as breads, cereals, and potatoes.

Certain plans require blind adherence to diets. They give little room for choice, or for meeting individual likes or dislikes.

Often diets are culturally-oriented and are geared only to the middle-class, white population.

The success of the local club depends to a large extent on the group leader and on his ability to generate interest and sustain motivation. If you're lucky, your group will have a dynamic leader.

Sometimes just being in a club sets up competition among the group members to lose weight fast. So what's wrong with that? Well, each person has his own metabolic rate, his own life style, his own needs, and should be privileged to set up his own rate of weight loss without excessive pressure.

Regular weigh-ins can encourage crash dieting each week just before the weigh-in. We have already pointed out how hard the body works to establish its own balance. It needn't be taxed unnecessarily by well-intentioned boomeranging procedures.

Not all clubs reeducate the dieter for intelligent, lifelong *self*-direction. If they did they would be putting themselves out of business.

The club can become a crutch to dieters—a security blanket. Once the initial stage of restored self-confidence is reached, you should be ready to take off on your own.

Leaders of groups are rarely trained nutritionists. They are usually former club members who have reached goal weight through the club's plan. Leaders receive propaganda training, but are not generally coached in the basics of nutrition or weight control principles. Misinformation is occasionally unintentionally passed on.

Leaders are not generally skilled or trained in counseling techniques. The group process sometimes leads to surprising self-analysis and disclosure. If emotional problems reveal themselves as a result of the diet or group process, the leader may find himself over his head.

Sometimes the plan can be too demanding and too pound-conscious. Short range plans seek immediate results and lack the perspective of long range plans. For example, the weigh-in may not make allowances for shifts in water balance during the menstrual cycle.

After being exposed to the basic series of lectures, the group member may tire of hearing the same lectures repeatedly. Boredom can quickly undermine motivation.

Most diet clubs tend to ignore the role of activity in weight control. Activity, if mentioned at all, is given only lip service. Profit-making clubs must focus on those weight control methods that will keep their dues-paying member coming back. Legal liability is also a deterrent. If a member were to increase his activity because of recommendations by the club and suffer some disorder as a consequence, the organization might find itself in legal difficulties. Thus the cardinal rule of management is generally: "Make no waves." Sometimes light exercises are done at the end of class. These are only mildly beneficial in developing tone or firming up muscle. Leaders and instructors are generally ignorant of the extremely important role activity can play in a sustained weight control program. Without regular, moderately vigorous activity, the successful diet club member may look thinner, but display flabby pouches of excess skin tissue.

CHARACTERISTICS OF VARIOUS CLUBS

If you are so minded, you will find that there is a wide choice of clubs. The following information will tell you about some of the basic differences that exist among the current alternatives.

There is also wide variation among local chapters of the same organization, due to geographic location, group membership, and group leadership. If you are not satisfied with your group or leader, you should consider transferring to another group or club. Most of the clubs, both profit and nonprofit, are interested in improving their effectiveness, and are trying new ideas. For example, behavior modification techniques are now being encouraged by most clubs' national headquarters.

The information which follows may have already undergone some change, especially in the dues structure.

Profit Making Organizations

A. *Weight Watchers International Incorporated*
   175 East Shore Road
   Great Neck, Long Island, New York 11023
   Telephone: (516) 466-5900

Weight Watchers, founded by Jean Nidetch in the mid-1960's and recently purchased by Pillsbury Company, has been enormously successful. Registration fees vary from $3.00 to $5.00, and weekly membership fees range from $2.00 to $4.00, depending on your geographic location. There are no penalty charges for gaining weight.

Weight Watchers estimates that five million people have contacted the organization since the program's inception, but information is not available on what percentage of that number may be composed of dropouts and repeaters.

At each meeting, the members, about fifty per class, weigh in, listen to a lecture or participate in a discussion about dieting and motivation, have an opportunity to ask questions, and spend some time socializing. The atmosphere is one of warmth and camaraderie.

The diet each weight watcher must follow is safe, workable and balanced. However, it is strict. Weight Watchers prescribes exactly what you may eat; no substitutions are allowed. There are different reducing diets for women (1200 calorie); men (1600 calorie); and adolescents. There are also leveling and maintenance plans for each of these three groups. Fish must be eaten at least five times a week and liver once a week. Alcohol is strictly forbidden.

Weight Watchers' chief drawbacks: Exercise is neither discouraged nor encouraged; and the group leaders are not as a rule adequately trained in nutrition or in counseling.

Weight Watchers is currently introducing skillful behavior modification techniques under the guidance of Dr. Richard Stuart, co-author of *Slim Chance in a Fat World,* Champaign: Research Press Company, 1972.

B. *The Diet Workshop Incorporated*
28 Merrick Avenue
Merrick, Long Island, New York 11566
Telephone: (516) 378-2510

Lois Lindauer, a former Weight Watcher, founded Diet Workshop in 1965 because she felt that the Weight Watchers plan was too rigid, and did not sufficiently consider the emotional needs of its members.

The fees include a $6.00 registration fee and a $2.50 weekly charge. There is a commitment plan that charges $25.00 for the first ten-week stint and goes down to $18.00 for subsequent ten-week sessions. A mini-loser plan—for those who want to lose ten pounds or less—is available for a flat fee of $15.00 for six weeks.

Weekly weigh-ins, lectures, discussions, mild isometric activities, followed by a social time comprise the meeting.

The Diet Workshop likes to be known as the program that cares. Its purpose is to help you reach goal weight and *stay* there. An excellent social program is available in some areas and includes such functions as a recipe contest; a "Ms. Diet Workshop" contest; and a yearly fashion show. These activities give the members a chance to appropriately show off and develop some long needed pride and self-confidence.

The diets are safe, balanced, and workable. However, diet workshoppers do not count calories. The diets are portion-controlled, with alcohol, rice, and potatoes forbidden. Nevertheless, this program has more flexibility than the traditional Weight Watchers plan.

If you enjoy talking about food, Diet Workshop may be your club. New recipes are offered weekly in class. Many cookbooks with tasty, supposedly low-calorie recipes are available for small fees.

Non-Profit Groups

A. TOPS
4575 South 5th Street
P. O. Box 4489
Milwaukee, Wisconsin 53207
Telephone: (414) 482-4620

TOPS, an acronym for "Take Off Pounds Sensibly," was founded in 1948 by Ester Manz. This non-profit, tax-exempt organization now has over 330,000 members throughout the world. In the year of 1971 they collectively lost 1.244 tons or about 2½ million pounds of weight.

TOPS has five distinguishing characteristics:

1. *Medical orientation.*   Members obtain their weight goals and their diets from their personal physicians.

2. *Psychotherapy orientation.*   Warm, personal support through phone calls, cards, letters, and personal visits sustain members between meetings. Although the order of business at chapter meetings varies, it usually includes a weigh-in and a talk or discussion on some phase of overweight. The program is quite social, with games, contests, sing-alongs, skits, and other forms of entertainment, all related to weight control. Each meeting begins with the recital of the TOPS pledge:

   I am an intelligent person. I will control my emotions, and not let my emotions control me. Every time I am tempted to use food to satisfy my frustrated desires, build up my injured ego, or dull my senses, I will remember even though I overeat in private my excess poundage is there for all the world to see. What a fool I've been.

3. *Competition.* Competition in weight loss at the chapter, area, state, and international levels is encouraged. Outstanding weight loss is rewarded with trophies, charms, and bracelets. Rallies and recognition days are organized on the state and national levels.

4. *Obesity Research* The membership fees for TOPS are quite nominal and some of these proceeds are set aside for an obesity and metabolic research program headquartered at Deaconess Hospital in Milwaukee, Wisconsin. Fee is $7.00 annually for the first two years, and $5.00 annually thereafter. Some local groups have an additional monthly fee of $.35 or less.

5. *Self-Direction* No diet is prescribed, since the founders of the group view this as an individual medical decision. Theoretically, this is the most sensible approach. However, it is less than perfect in practice because of the poor nutritional education of many medical practitioners. The sensible shedding of excessive fat is subject to the ideas, whims, and fancies of the physician. The diets of some members may or may not be workable, safe, or balanced, depending on the physician prescribing them.

B. *Overeaters Anonymous*
   P. O. Box 2613
   Hollywood, Calif. 90028
   Telephone: (213) 475-8654

Overeaters Anonymous
World Service Office
3730 Motor Avenue
Los Angeles, Calif. 90034
Telephone: (213) 559-6140

Founded in 1960, Overeaters Anonymous (O. A.) is patterned after Alcoholics Anonymous. Meetings open with the A. A. prayer of serenity: "God grant me the serenity to accept the things I cannot change; the courage to change the things I can; and the wisdom to know the difference." The meetings close with a recital of the Lord's Prayer, with all the members holding hands.

Overeaters Anonymous describes itself as "a fellowship of men and women who have a common problem—compulsive eating. They have joined together to share their experience, strength, and hope with one another in order to solve this problem and to help other compulsive eaters to do the same."

Like the highly successful A.A. program, the group attracts people who need other people and who need to rely on a power outside themselves to control their compulsive consumption. Many O.A. members first went the route of all the other diet clubs and then found what they needed in O.A. membership. These compulsive eaters have one thing in common: they are driven by forces they don't understand to eat more than they need. This compulsive consumption is often binge eating. O.A. helps break this pattern by suggesting that members call each other on the telephone when tempted, or call on the Higher Power for strength.

Rather than looking ahead to the future, members are encouraged to take one day at a time. The OA mottos are as follows:

JUST FOR TODAY I will try to live through this day only, and not tackle my whole life problem at once. I can do something for twelve hours that would appall me if I felt that I had to keep it up for a lifetime.

JUST FOR TODAY I will be happy. This assumes to be true what Abraham Lincoln said, that "most folks are as happy as they make up their minds to be."

JUST FOR TODAY I will exercise my soul in three ways: I will do somebody a good turn and not get found out; if anybody knows of it, it will not count. I will do at least two things I don't want to do—just for exercise. I will not show anyone that my feelings are hurt; they may be hurt, but today I will not show it.

JUST FOR TODAY I will be agreeable. I will look as well as I can, dress becomingly, talk low, act courteously, criticize not one bit, not find fault with anything and not try to improve or regulate anybody except myself.

JUST FOR TODAY I will have a program. I may not follow it exactly, but I will have it. I will save myself from two pests: hurry and indecision.

JUST FOR TODAY I will have a quiet half hour all by myself, and relax. During this half hour, some time, I will try to get a better perspective on my life.

JUST FOR TODAY I will be unafraid. Especially I will not be afraid to enjoy what is beautiful, and to *believe that as I give to the world, so the world will give to me.**

Overeaters Anonymous charges no dues; it supports itself through the voluntary contributions of its members. Talk about food is discouraged; emphasis is on the psychotherapeutic value of the group. No diets are prescribed, but guidelines are given. For example, members interested in special diets are strongly advised to consult their personal physicians. O.A.'s psychological approach is excellent.

The Carboholic Strainer Theory

Carbohydrates—sugar and starches—are said to be the downfall of many a conscientious dieter. The ingestion of the smallest quantity of carbohydrates seems to trigger a reflex mechanism which signals the eater to go on a binge comparable to that of the alcoholic. This disease has been referred to as "carboholism"—rendering one's life unmanageable as a result of ingesting excessive quantities of carbohydrate foods.

Now picture within each person a strainer, whose function it is to gradually filter carbohydrates through the metabolic process. If the strainer becomes faulty or breaks down, the amount of carbohydrates released into the system becomes overwhelming. Paradoxically, this flooding of the system triggers carboholism—the abnormal reaction to consume even more carbohydrates.

The strainer, once ruptured, will probably never repair itself. Therefore, it is necessary for carboholics to avoid their

* Permission granted by Overeaters Anonymous, Box 34854, Los Angeles, Calif. 90034

particular binge foods—one day at a time—for the rest of their lives.

Speculation based on the Strainer Theory suggests that overexposure to refined carbohydrates, such as those empty calories of junk foods, debilitates the strainer before its time.

Some persons may have inherited a weak strainer which breaks down early in life. Others, by continually bombarding the strainer with carbohydrates, eventually will destroy their strainers.

1. What condition would you say *your* strainer is in?

2. List five foods that have binge potential in your life. Rank order them.

Rank   **Food**

———————   ————————————

———————   ————————————

———————   ————————————

———————   ————————————

———————   ————————————

Circle those that are predominantly carbohydrates or refined sugars.

3. What alternatives could you use to control binge consumption of these foods?

4. Circle the most reasonable of the above alternatives?

5. What course of action do you feel you can establish in order to deal with your binge eating?

SUMMARY OF DIET CLUBS

Weight Watchers is a profit-making organization offering a well-balanced diet and an excellent all-round program.

Diet Workshop is a profit-making organization providing some flexibility in diet and a social atmosphere. It too has an excellent diet program.

TOPS is a nonprofit social organization with a diet plan supplied by each member's personal physician. Emphasis is on emotional strength and self-direction.

Overeaters Anonymous is a nonprofit organization that helps you abstain from compulsive eating of binge foods while you get yourself together emotionally and psychologically.

What You Know May Not Be So

The noted Harvard nutritionist, Jean Mayer, has said, "Scientific research is changing our ideas all the time. We not only keep learning new things we didn't know before, but we also have to unlearn things we thought we knew, but now turn out not to be so."[1]

Of all the scientists who ever lived, 90% are alive and doing research today. As a partial consequence of all this research, some of the sciences are experiencing a doubling of knowledge every ten years. In addition to the 60,000,000 pages of scientific and technical literature published each year, there are over one thousand new books rolling off printing presses each day![2] All this has created a knowledge explosion of unprecedented magnitude. Even a proficient speed reader has difficulty keeping abreast of new findings within his field of specialization.

One aspect of this knowledge explosion is that once-accepted facts are now being questioned. Truth, once relatively constant, has taken on a half-life of believability because of new scientific discoveries. We live in a time when answering questions is not enough; now we are not satisfied unless we are also questioning old answers.

In a society where "yesterday's truths suddenly become today's fictions"[3], we should all periodically reevaluate our knowledge. Most readers would recognize the inaccuracy of once-accepted statements like these:

Eating bread crusts will make your hair curly.

Eating meat more than once a day is harmful.

Wine makes blood.

Eating prunes will prevent wrinkles.

An apple a day keeps the doctor away.

Thunder and lightning will cause milk to sour.

Many of these old wives' tales are snickered at today because of the level of knowledge that we have attained. However, even today "there are possibly more misconceptions and half-truths still believed by the American public in nutrition than in any other area of health."[4]

Up-to-date information is a necessary ingredient of a successful weight control program. If you are to base your behavior on current information and theories, then you would be wise to check on the accuracy of your nutrition knowledge. As the late Ernie Pyle once said, "It ain't the things you don't know that make you a fool; it's the things you know that ain't so."

The following quiz is designed to uncover nutritional misconceptions—practices or beliefs that are not in accord with the latest scientific information. The answers and discussion will be found at the end of the test.

Nutrition and Weight Control Knowledge Test

Directions: Circle T or F if you think the statement is true or false. If you are not sure of the correct answer, circle DK—"don't know." You may wish to jot notes in the margin to justify your answers and check them out with the explanations which follow the quiz.

T F DK   1. It is dangerous to leave food in an open tin can in the refrigerator.

T F DK   2. A daily bowel movement is necessary for good health.

T F DK   3. A well-trained athlete needs the same amount of protein as a less active person of the same weight, sex, and age.

T F DK   4. Gelatin is one of the best sources of protein.

T F DK   5. There are living bacteria in pasteurized milk.

T F DK   6. Milk contains all the essential elements of a good diet and in sufficient quantities to insure good health and normal body development.

T F DK   7. The average American can prevent colds by taking vitamin pills.

T F DK   8. Inexpensive meats are just as nutritious as expensive meats.

T F DK   9. Women in their childbearing years need more iron than men.

T F DK   10. Give a child all the food he wants and he will never suffer from malnutrition.

T F DK   11. Polyunsaturated fats are lower in calories than saturated fats.

T F DK   12. Potatoes are a fattening food.

T F DK   13. Margarine contains fewer calories than butter.

T F DK   14. Dark bread has about the same caloric value as white bread.

T F DK   15. Most people are overweight because of the fattening types of food they consume, rather than the amount they eat.

T F DK   16. You don't gain weight from meat because meat burns its own calories.

T F DK   17. Toasted bread has significantly fewer calories than untoasted bread.

T F DK   18. Glandular trouble is the major cause of obesity.

T F DK   19. Vitamins and minerals yield no calories.

T F DK   20. Once a person stops exercising, muscle fibers change to fat.

T F DK   21. Eating grapefruit with your regular meals will help you reduce.

T F DK   22. Alcohol contains more calories per gram than starches.

T F DK   23. Fruits and fruit juices can be fattening if consumed in excess of your total caloric need.

T F DK   24. High protein foods such as meat and fish contain practically no calories.

T F DK   25. Even if you take reducing pills, you still cannot eat all you want and expect to lose weight.

Answers

The above questions were part of a larger test given to over 1,300 college freshmen at a large Eastern university.[5] Below are the correct responses. Beside each correct answer is the percentage of these college students that gave the correct answer.

1.	False	16%	4.	False	26%
2.	False	18%	5.	True	31%
3.	True	18%	6.	False	51%

7.	False	75%	17.	False	39%
8.	True	82%	18.	False	41%
9.	True	91%	19.	True	42%
10.	False	91%	20.	False	45%
11.	False	12%	21.	False	46%
12.	False	13%	22.	True	51%
13.	False	13%	23.	True	57%
14.	True	18%	24.	False	66%
15.	False	25%	25.	True	85%
16.	False	38%			

Evaluation Scale

23-25 correct — Excellent; you must teach nutrition.

20-22 correct — Good; you have done some reading.

18-19 correct — Average; you have a general knowledge of nutrition.

15-17 correct — Fair; you had better reevaluate your source of information.

14 or less correct — Read on, and on, and on.

Discussion of Quiz Answers

Below are explanations of the correct quiz answers. Read all the explanations, including those for the questions you got right, to make sure you understand the principles involved. Remember, what you don't know may hurt you.

1. It is not dangerous to leave food in an open tin can in the refrigerator. The U.S. Department of Agriculture states that it is safe to keep food in the original can after it has been opened. It is important to cover the can and to keep

the food cool. A few acid foods may dissolve a little tin from the can, but this is not harmful or dangerous to one's health.

2. It is not necessary to have a bowel movement every day. Each person establishes his own pattern of elimination based on many factors: his ingestion of foods high in roughage and fiber content (e.g. raw vegetables); his activity level; his individual biochemical makeup, which differs from person to person; and his natural body rhythms. Elimination every other day or even every third day is considered within the realm of normality. There is evidence, however, that diets low in fiber content increase the likelihood of cancer of the colon and rectum.

3. Even though certain protein-pill manufacturers would like athletes—especially weight lifters—to believe otherwise, athletes have no special need for extra protein. As a rule of thumb, nùtritionists recommend about .45 grams of protein per day per pound of body weight for adults. Growing children need at least twice that amount. The average American adult consumes almost three times the recommended amount of protein per day, athletes even more.

4. Gelatin is not an excellent source of protein, since it does not contain all of the essential amino acids necessary for growth, repair, and maintenance of the body. Nor has it been conclusively demonstrated that gelatin can keep the finger nails from becoming too brittle. The original research on this was carried out by a company that produces gelatin. Their research has never been replicated; researchers have not felt this notion important

enough to check out the claims of the manufacturer.

As a rule of thumb, no *one* food has any special health-giving qualities; it is one's total nutrient intake that affects the overall health of the organism.

5. During pasteurization the temperature of milk is raised to over 160° Fahrenheit for a short period of time. This process kills off only those bacteria that would cause disease in man. Milk spoils because of the remaining bacteria which, as they increase in number, eat the milk sugar (lactose) and give off a waste product that gives spoiled milk its characteristic odor.

6. Milk is not a perfect food. It is low in iron and low in vitamin C (ascorbic acid). Milk, however, does contain a variety of necessary nutrients in fairly large quantities, particularly calcium. When used as recommended, milk, and milk products—cheese, ice cream, and yogurt—contribute substantially to a proper diet.

7. There is not enough evidence to conclude that colds can be prevented by taking vitamin pills, even though some well-intentioned scientists would have you believe otherwise. The preventive and even curative powers of vitamin C (claimed by Linus Pauling, who won his Nobel prize in another field) have not been proven to the satisfaction of nutrition researchers.

Another nutritional rule of thumb: You *can* have too much of a good thing. Excesses of vitamin A and vitamin D can produce poisonous effects, since these nutrients are stored in fat tissues. Vitamin C, however, is not stored in the body; once the tissues are replete, the excess intake is excreted. Therefore, more than six ounces of orange juice on any given day is nothing but an expensive source of urine. The extremely high dosages of vitamin C that have been recommended to prevent and cure colds can cause kidney damage in susceptible persons, particularly if the water ingestion of the pill-popper is low, creating a more concentrated vitamin C level for the kidneys to process and excrete. Also, taking in large quantities of vitamin C interferes with the absorption of vitamin B-12. Remember *quid pro quo*— "something in exchange for something"? The body functions best in balance—medically called homeostasis.

8. Inexpensive meats may be just as nutritious as expensive meats. Meat is meat. It contains complete protein—that is, all eight essential amino acids—and it matters not whether the meat is an expensive cut or a less expensive one. Regardless of the cost of the meat, you should routinely drain or trim off excess fat before eating it.

9. Women in their childbearing years do need more iron than men. This is due primarily to the monthly loss of iron at menstruation, and also to their special needs during pregnancy. As you may have noted, only 9% of the college students tested scored wrong on this question. No doubt the public has been "educated" by the half-truths of vitamin-plus-iron advertisements.

10. Given unlimited choice children will invariably choose sweet food. The child has no built-in mechanism of craving foods he needs. Even obese children suffer from malnutrition, so quantity is no guarantee of quality.

11. Saturated and polyunsaturated fats have the same number of calories. Saturated fats come from animal sources and coconut oil. Most of them are solid at room temperature and contain appreciable amounts of cholesterol.

Chemically, a saturated fat is a completed chain; there are no open links—called double bonds—where hydrogen can be added to the chain. Unsaturated fats generally are of a vegetable origin, liquid at room temperature, and contain no cholesterol. Unsaturated fats have one or more double bonds where hydrogen can be added. The polyunsaturated fat has two or more places where hydrogen can be added. Adding hydrogen to certain unsaturated fats renders them semisolid at room temperature, so that they do not become rancid as rapidly as other fats.

12. Potatoes are *not* overly fattening. Most people use the following logic, called syllogistic reasoning: Potatoes are starch; starch is fattening; therefore, potatoes are fattening. The logic is good, but the premise that starch is fattening is incorrect and therefore the deduction is incorrect.

Fattening is a relative term. It must be judged in terms of one's total calorie intake in relation to one's total calorie expenditure. By definition, no one food is fattening, in and of itself. On the other hand, any calorie-containing food can become fattening if eaten in excess of one's total daily need.

Some foods—like ice cream—have high calorie contents, but taken in small quantities ice cream has far fewer calories than the average serving of meat. Three ounces of sirloin steak can range from 175 calories (lean meat) to 330 calories (more fatty meat). An average serving of one sixth of a quart of chocolate ice cream (approximately three ounces) contains 200 calories. A smaller-than-average serving of two ounces of chocolate ice cream has a caloric content of under 135. Of course, the danger with ice cream is that it can become a binge food. But in moderation, ice cream, like potatoes, needn't be unduly "fattening."

A medium-large baked potato contains about 100 calories *without butter or sour cream*. Like sugar, starch is a carbohydrate and contains four calories per gram. Protein must be just as fattening because protein also contains four calories per gram. Alcohol contains seven calories per gram, and fat nine—making these twice as fattening as starch. Starch is far from the most fattening caloric source available.

If starch is so fattening, then those whose diet is predominantly starch should be the fattest people on earth. But this is not the case. Rice is a starch food; yet as a rule, the thinnest populations in the world are those whose staple—and sometimes only—food is rice. The reason they are not fat should be obvious—they do not eat rice or any other food in excess of their total daily needs. Most of the rice-consuming nations don't have enough of this "fattening" food—or any other—to cause even mild overweight, let alone obesity.

13. Margarine and butter contain the same number of calories per gram. Margarine generally comes from a vegetable source, butter from an animal source. The two are identical, nutritionally speaking, except that butter contains a sizable amount of cholesterol while vegetable-oil margarines contain none.

Don't be fooled by diet margarines. They claim fewer calories per serving than regular margarines, but by weight of the product *without fillers* the calorie content is similar. Some manufacturers inject air into their margarine to justify the claim of fewer calories per volume; noncaloric fillers are used by other companies.

In the end, margarine must always be made from oils and nothing can be done to reduce the nine calories per gram that oil contains.

14. White bread—sixty-four calories per slice, and whole wheat bread—fifty-seven calories per slice—are very similar in caloric value. Other breads do have a wider range of caloric content. For example, one slice of Boston brown bread contains ninety-six calories, but it makes up for its calories in nutritional quality.

15. As stated earlier, no food, in and of itself, can be considered fattening. It is the total calorie intake—usually reflected in the total amount people eat—in relation to one's need that determines whether or not a person will gain weight. Most overweight people eat too much—of all foods, including the so-called fattening kinds—and exercise too little.

16. Meat does not burn its own calories. Some weight control programs emphasize the importance of a high protein intake on the grounds that meat creates within the body a higher specific dynamic action (S.D.A.) than other foods, and that this S.D.A. reduces the total number of excess calories that can be converted into fat. However, what these meat faddists fail to tell you is that the S.D.A. quotient has already been taken into account when protein is assessed at four calories per gram. Meat is generally interlaced with fat—visible or invisible—and fat is the *most* concentrated source of calories. Contrary to popular belief, meat products have the *highest* caloric content per serving compared to the other three food groups.

17. Toasted bread has the same number of calories as un-

toasted bread, provided not too many crumbs have fallen off the bread as it is being toasted. There is a difference in the moisture content, but since there are no calories in water, the calorie content of the bread remains unchanged.

18. The major cause of obesity is not glandular, but due to the consumption over a given period of time of more calories than the body requires. With an underactive thyroid gland the body burns fewer calories. A person with a hypoactive thyroid gland, then, needs fewer calories to get through the day than a person with a normal thyroid. If the person with the underactive gland tries to match calories with a person whose thyroid is normal, the former will gain weight because *his* intake is exceeding *his* needs.

19. Vitamins and minerals are consumed in such a small quantity that even if they did yield calories, their contribution would be insignificant. The sum weight of all the vitamins needed per day only amounts to 1/237th of an ounce.

20. When a person stops exercising, muscle fibers lose their tone and decrease in size and weight. An increase in activity combined with a decrease in total calorie intake can reverse this process.

21. There appears to be no magic instant formula that will help people reduce. The only magic combination is balancing your total calorie intake with your total calorie expenditure.

22. Alcohol does not contain more calories per gram than starches. In fact, alcohol takes priority in your system—

the calories from alcohol must be used up *before* the calories from other foods stored in the blood stream can be utilized.

23.   Any food—even something as good for you as fruit juices—eaten in excess of your total needs has the potential to become "fattening." Nutritious foods are no exception.

24.   The Meat Group is generally high in calories because the meat is interlaced with fat. Fish is generally low in fat and high in protein, but it still contains calories. When our protein and nitrogen needs are met, the body converts excess protein calories into fat for storage, just as it would excess calories from any source except alcohol. The body does not discriminate as to the source of calories it converts to fat.

25.   The various types of reducing pills only moderately increase the metabolic rate, decrease the appetite, or eliminate excess fluids. They are chiefly intended to give a person chemical help in maintaining his motivation on a weight control plan by depressing his appetite. If you eat more than you need you will gain weight even with pills. Pills cannot replace a weight control plan based on calorie reduction and activity increase.

EFFECTS OF MISINFORMATION

Believing some of the untrue statements in the quiz could be hazardous to your health. If, for example, you believed that meat burned its own calories and therefore kept to a diet high in meat products, the excess calories could show up around your waist in the form of adipose tissue—which is to say, *fat*.

Often, information absorbed early in life interferes with the learning of accurate information later on. Educational psychologists call this phenomenon "proactive inhibition." This means that once you've learned something incorrect, it takes more than twice as much effort to learn the correct information. For example, you must first *un*learn the misconception that potatoes are fattening. Then you can start to *re*learn that starch and protein have the same number of calories per gram, and that fattening is a relatively meaningless word in isolation.

If new information conflicts with your previously held beliefs, you may find it hard to absorb. This phenomenon, referred to as cognitive dissonance, accounts for a person's normal resistance to change. Over time, with continued reinforcement, the more accurate information will replace the misinformation. Eventually the new information may be absorbed on a behavioral level. Change is a gradual process and it may take months to actualize new information in your behavior.

But, as John Locke once wrote, "The actions of men are the best interpreters of their thoughts." Once you are really convinced that, for example, potatoes are not necessarily fattening, or that activity is crucial in weight loss, you won't hesitate to make room for these concepts in your life pattern.

SOURCES OF MISINFORMATION

Old wives' tales have been handed down from generation to generation; rarely do we double-check them for accuracy.

A more subtle and possibly more effective source of misinformation are the half-truths propagated by the media. Products are advertised to increase sales. If this means stretching the truth, then the truth generally is stretched; often it means telling only part of the truth. Vitamin pills are a waste of money for the person who follows the Four Food Groups, yet the ad men persuade people that they ought to take vitamins anyway—just to be sure. Dieters often buy diet bread because it is advertised as having fewer calories per slice. While this fact is true, the *whole* truth is that the diet bread contains no special low-calorie ingredients; it's usually regular bread sliced thinner!

Some food manufacturers take advantage of the general ignorance about nutrition to sway the public to their point of view. They are often aided by food faddists who are generally skilled in persuasive techniques and have the knack of telling people what they want to hear. Caught up in the zeal of the faddist, and lacking any information of their own on the subject, many otherwise intelligent consumers become convinced of the need for certain so-called health foods. In reality, there is no such thing as a "health food." Most foods have certain health giving properties, some foods more than others. Generally, a scare tactic of some sort is used, and pseudoscientific books and journals are often quoted. The reader rarely checks the references. Most of the statements are impossible to prove, but they are also extremely difficult to disprove. Their generalizations should be carefully investigated and not accepted as unquestionable gospel.

SOME MYTHS ABOUT NUTRITION

As the food industry has become big business, there has been a growing concern that advanced technological and scientific techniques have rendered our food supplies less pure. It is healthy to be skeptical and examine carefully what you are being urged to consume. But, by the same token, it is advisable to be wary of nutritional myths spread by some alarmists. Here are four common ones to avoid.

1. *Most diseases are caused by a faulty diet.*

    Of course *some* diseases—goiter, anemia, rickets, and certain forms of heart disease—can be triggered by poor diet. However, many other diseases are caused by heredity, birth defects, the aging process, and poor health habits such as excessive smoking or overconsumption of alcohol. As Adelle Davis's death demonstrated, the most nutrition-conscious individuals may fall prey to diseases largely beyond their control.

2. *The American soil is being impoverished and produces food that is inferior in nutritional value.*

    Promoters of this myth also attack chemical fertilizers as being poisonous. It is not generally known that the majority of the nutritive components of a fruit or vegetable come from the quality of the seed, not the soil. Given a minimally healthy environment, the seed will grow to harvest as nature intended, regardless of the type of fertilizer used. The soil breaks down the fertilizer—whether it be natural or chemical—into basic building blocks of carbon, hydrogen, and oxygen. The plant really doesn't seem to care what source these basics originally came from. Fertilizers—whether chemical or natural—do little to alter the quality of the plant; they only affect quantity—the yield per acre. Organically fertilized foods have not been shown to be either superior or inferior to chemically fertilized foods. The only difference shown thus far is that chemicals result in larger, faster yields per acre. Organic fertilizers may have some minerals and elements not present in chemical fertilizers, but this remains to be proved. What is true is that organically fertilized soil retains more moisture than soil repeatedly fertilized with chemicals.

One disease—simple goiter—has been associated with soil deficiency—the absence or low concentration of iodine in the soil. Today one's need for this essential nutrient is usually fulfilled by the use of iodized salt.

While we all tend to be wary of large-scale meddling with nature, more often than not scientific intervention has improved the quality of life. Without the use of pesticides, crop failure due to insect blight can cause millions to go unfed. Of course pesticides should be used more judiciously, and careful consumer washing of produce is recommended.

3. *The American food supply is devitalized by overprocessing.*

Promoters of special cookware and of dietary supplements would like to convince the public of this myth to help increase sales. White enriched breads often come under attack. A common assertion is that the milling process robs wheat of twenty important nutrients, of which only four are put back. True, processed, bleached white flour lacks the nutritional germ and bran of whole wheat. But recent research has indicated that a substance found in whole-wheat flour—phytates—may impede the body's absorption of the iron found in wheat.[6] Enriched white flour contains thiamin, riboflavin, niacin, and iron, but no phytates. However, whole wheat bread does contribute importantly to the body's fiber needs and provides other nutrients in small amounts. Variety in the selection of products increases the probability of meeting one's nutritional needs.

Criticism has also centered on the many additives found in the American food supply. These chemical additives, which attempt to preserve freshness and flavor, are "Generally Recognized as Safe" (GRAS) by the Food and Drug Administration. However, even though additives have not been proven harmful, the cautious individual may wish to minimize his ingestion of *any* nonnutritive substance, since no one can be sure what the long range effects will be.

4. *Most Americans suffer from subclinical deficiencies of needed vitamins and minerals, and should take vitamin-mineral supplements and eat health foods to insure good health.*

According to this myth, if you have that tired, run-down feeling you probably suffer from subclinical deficiencies. The promoters of food supplements state that since these deficiencies cannot be measured or evaluated by known clinical procedures a person is well-advised to take their specially-designed concoctions—just in case. And so the food supplement industry reaps the profits of a multi-billion-dollar business.

As has been pointed out earlier, there are certain deficiencies characteristic of the American diet. But these can easily be counteracted through sensible eating.

WHAT CAN YOU DO
ABOUT MISINFORMATION

To protect yourself against fraudulent schemes and unnecessary products a certain amount of basic knowledge is needed. Your orientation should be factual, but with emphasis on grasping the basic principles of nutrition. In this way you can use these underlying concepts—which probably won't change—as a yardstick to measure the accuracy of new information or misinformation.

Have you ever caught yourself saying, "Gee, that's complicated, but I guess if I don't understand it, it must be true"? Some advertisers, food faddists, and quacks capitalize on consumers' ignorance. A better rule to follow is: "I won't buy it because I don't understand it." Be skeptical, especially if someone is after your money. Armed with the basic nutritional concepts, you will be better protected as you fight the war of "caveat emptor"—*let the consumer beware.*

Stop believing everything you read. (Yes, that includes this book.) Begin to question assumptions. A "prove it to me" skepticism may be the appropriate attitude to adopt in matters concerning money and health. College graduates tend to believe more of what they read in print than high school graduates, and high school graduates more than high school dropouts. Most of us have forgotten that, in the interests of protecting freedom of the press, the Constitution does not prevent authors and publishers from distorting the truth, or even lying in print. You yourself should check out information before you act on it.

GUIDELINES FOR EVALUATING NUTRITION AND WEIGHT CONTROL INFORMATION

To evaluate the reliability of information, you should be concerned about its accuracy, completeness and relevance to the topic. Is the information being disseminated designed to protect vested interests? What are the goals or intents of the author?

Find out what qualifies the author to write the book or article. What makes him an authority in this field? Has he done research or study in this area? Has the author been trained in a good program at a recognized university? What is the author's experience in nutrition education or research? Does he currently belong to learned societies and organizations related to the subject about which he is writing?

Don't be overly impressed by an author's academic degrees. As convincing as these degrees may seem, they only indicate that the author has endured more schooling than the average person. A degree does not assure the reader that the author is knowledgeable about the subject of the book. Some people have expertise in more than one field; however, many so-called "experts" in one field write about subjects on which they have less knowledge, hoping their authority will carry over.

Check to see whether the author holds a degree in the field about which he is writing. Linus Pauling, the Nobel Peace Prize winner in physics, wrote *Vitamin C and The Common Cold*. As impressive as are his credentials in physics, he is not a "recognized" authority in the field of nutrition.

Be skeptical when an author quotes research, especially if he doesn't give you the reference. Research can be misquoted and is often misinterpreted. Be wary of generalizations in research findings. Research doesn't really prove anything. Be careful not to get sucked into believing any statement that begins, "Studies have proven that . . . " Research, at best, can only support or not support a hypothesis. In and of itself, one study cannot be definitive. Research design is usually so carefully delineated, so narrow in scope that it can only contribute a small piece of information to the general body of knowledge and formation of theories. Quoting statistics can sometimes be a trick. Be careful of how numbers are used, especially if a correlation is being made between two sets of data. Reliable studies are generally cautious in their conclusions and avoid sweeping statements, generalizations, or implications about causality.

Beware of the persecution complex of some authors. Often they will state, "I am being persecuted by large medical trusts and organizations. They attack what I am writing because they have vested interests to protect. They refute what I write because they would otherwise lose hundreds of thousands of dollars." This ploy is often used by quacks pushing anything from special cancer cures to vitamin supplements. You will have to judge for yourself the author's credibility.

AT LEAST KNOW WHAT "AIN'T SO"

Knowledge is perhaps your best safeguard against the modern day medicine man. Fortify yourself with the basic concepts of calorie balance, the Four Food Groups, and the principles of weight control.

W. D. Forsythe, agreeing with Ernie Pyle, suggests that it is frequently "not ignorance alone that matters, but knowing so much that is not so."[7] He tells about a steamboat pilot who was asked if he knew where all the protruding rocks and boat snags were in the river. The pilot replied that he did not know where they all were, but he knew "where they ain't."

This is aptly applied to misconceptions about food. You can never hope to keep abreast of all of the latest scientific research in the field of nutrition, but you can at least know what "ain't so."

REFERENCES

1. Engel, Mary Jane, and Mae Rudolph, "Let's Talk about Good Foods," *Family Health,* vol. II, no. 7, July, 1970, p. 26.

2. Toffler, Alvin, *Future Shock,* New York: Random House, 1970, pp. 30, 31.

3. *Ibid.,* p. 140.

4. Kilander, H.F. "The Public's Belief in Nutrition Facts and Fallacies," *Journal of School Health,* Vol. 34, May 1964, p. 220.

5. Osman, Jack D. and Richard A. Ahrens, "Nutrition Misconceptions of College Freshmen," *School Health Review,* Nov.-Dec., 1972.

6. Stare, F. J., and M. McWilliams, *Living Nutrition,* New York: John Wiley and Sons, Inc., 1973, p. 334.

7. Forsythe, W. D., "Thirty-one Fallacies About Health," *Hygeia,* 25 July, 1947: 512.

Resolving Some Confusions

You have absorbed tons of information on nutrition and dieting and activity; you're rarin' to go; you want to put your newly acquired resolution and knowledge into practice. And now you find yourself plagued by minute, practical questions. Let's see if we can work them out.

When I'm on a diet how many meals should I eat per day?
The same number of meals you have always eaten per day under normal circumstances. Many people drastically change their eating patterns in an attempt to reduce, only to revert to their old habits once they reach their desired weight. The important thing is to avoid consuming more calories over a given period of time than your body needs, whether you are eating those calories in one meal per day or spreading them out in six meals.

Our society has established three meals per day as the most efficient, effective, and satisfying eating pattern. For most people the breakfast, lunch, dinner pattern provides the needed breaks in the daily routine and time to socialize. Erratic eating patterns can cause difficulty for dieters. Establishing patterns in your eating behavior makes it easier to balance your food selection according to the Four Food Groups.

Smaller, more frequent meals are often recommended for dieters (e.g., diabetics) who need to keep something in their stomachs. This is fine provided the total calorie intake doesn't rise with the number of meals. More frequent feedings may establish a dangerous precedent when the person goes off his particular dietary regimen.

Conversely, eating only once or twice a day may make it difficult to ingest all of the appropriate nutrients recommended within the Four Food Groups. The importance of a good breakfast has already been pointed out. If you eat one meal per day, you run the risk of having an inadequate blood sugar supply with which to meet emergency situations and you may be subject to the concomitant fatigue resulting from a low blood sugar level.

Does eating at night, just before going to bed, cause a weight gain?

Generally, no. The total number of calories consumed over a twenty-four hour period compared to the total number of calories utilized by the body over the same period is the criterion for determining excessive calories. It does not matter when these calories are ingested. People assume that because fewer calories are burned in sleeping, the meal before bedtime stays with you. This is not necessarily so.

Vigorous daytime physical activity carries over to the evening metabolic rate. If you're very active during the day, you can burn calories even while you sleep.

On three meals a day I often get hungry during the evening hours. What should I do?

Believe it or not, hunger is something that few of us have ever experienced. Hunger means that the body has a physiological need for food. You would have to eat nothing at all for several days before feeling a real hunger pang. What most of us experience is *appetite*, or a craving for food, often brought on by reaction to cues such as the sight, smell, or thought of food. Unlike hunger, appetite is easily triggered and can be provoked by the subtle suggestions of advertising media. Despite all our diet consciousness, snacking has become part of the American life style. Rather than attempt to change this style, I suggest that you use it to your nutritional advantage.

Listed below are suggested snack foods. To benefit from snacking, you must plan ahead. Make a shopping list and stick to it. In the store everything looks good. A prudent selection of snack foods can supplement the nutritional foundation of the Four Food Groups. At least it will keep you away from snacks that will sabotage your weight control program. Remember, it's the totals that count.

Avoid candy and pastry snacking. Save these for very special occasions.

Snack Ideas

Cubes of cheese on picks

Cheese and crackers

Fresh fruit*

Meat cubes on picks*

Fruit salad

Carrot and celery sticks

Hard boiled eggs*

Radishes

Dry unsweetened cereal

Fresh vegetable wedges and cheese

Fresh fruit or berries with milk or cheese

Peanuts or peanut butter*

Sunflower seeds, pumpkin seeds

Yogurt

Cottage cheese

Leftovers of meat or fish*

Tuna

Cream cheese on date nut bread

Lunchmeats

*good sources of iron

Nuts of all kinds*

Coconut

Ice cream and ice milk

Cheese toast

Pizza

Prunes, Raisins, Apricots, Dates, Figs*

Molasses on bread*

Should I take vitamin pills while dieting?

The vitamin pill industry is a multimillion-dollar business. The public's dependence on vitamins is a need that has been created by successful advertising. Despite what you have been told by the media, vitamin pills are unnecessary for the overwhelming majority of the people who are using them. Some commercials do actually state that if you eat properly, vitamin pills are not really necessary. However, they then capitalize on the nutritional ignorance of the consumer by asking, "But how do you know if you are eating all the foods you should? Just to be sure, shouldn't you be taking Brand X Vitamin pills?"

If you are relatively healthy and are following the Four Food Groups, vitamin pills are a waste of money. The Four Food Groups will supply your body with all of the vitamins necessary to maintain your health.

If you pay close attention to advertising you will begin to note that the more a product is advertised, the less necessary for existence that product really is; the fewer differences there are among various brands of that product; and the more expensive the product is to the consumer. Vitamin pills are no exception. Even on a weight reduction diet, vitamin pills are unnecessary for the average, healthy American.

The vitamin chart below gives the important functions of each vitamin and the most readily-available sources of these vitamins.

VITAMIN CHART*

VITAMIN	IMPORTANT FUNCTIONS	IMPORTANT SOURCES
Vitamin A	Helps keep skin clear and smooth Helps keep mucous membranes firm and resistant to infection Helps prevent night blindness Promotes growth	Liver, yolk of egg Dark green and deep yellow vegetables Deep yellow fruits, as cantaloupe Butter, whole milk, cream cheese, ice cream
Thiamine	Helps promote normal appetite and digestion Helps keep nervous system healthy and prevent irritability Helps body obtain energy from food	Meat, fish, poultry—pork supplies about 3 times as much as other meats Eggs Enriched or whole grain bread and cereals Dried beans and peas Potatoes, broccoli, collards
Niacin	Helps keep nervous system healthy Helps keep skin, mouth, tongue, digestive tract in healthy condition Helps cells of the body use oxygen to produce energy	Peanut butter Meat, fish, poultry Milk (high in tryptophan) Enriched or whole grain breads and cereals
Ascorbic Acid or Vitamin C	Helps make cementing materials that hold body cells together Strengthens walls of blood vessels Helps in healing wounds and broken bones Helps teeth and bone formation	Citrus fruits—orange, grapefruit, lemon, lime Strawberries and cantaloupe Tomatoes Green peppers, broccoli Greens, cabbage Potatoes
Vitamin D The Sunshine Vitamin	Helps body use calcium and phosphorus to build strong bones and teeth	Vitamin D milk Fish liver oils Sunshine on skin (not a food)
Riboflavin	Helps cells use oxygen to release energy from foods Helps keep skin, tongue and lips normal Helps prevent scaly, greasy skin around mouth and nose	Milk, cheese, ice cream Meat, especially liver Fish, poultry and eggs
Vitamin B_6	Helps nervous tissues function normally Plays a role in red cell regeneration Involved in the metabolism of amino acids, fats and carbohydrates	Beef liver, pork and ham Soybeans and lima beans Bananas Yeast Whole grain cereals
Vitamin B_{12}	Protects against the development of pernicious anemia	Eggs, fish, liver and other meat Milk

*Courtesy of the Milk Foundation, Chicago

VITAMIN	IMPORTANT FUNCTIONS	IMPORTANT SOURCES
Vitamin E	In lower animals, maintains normal functioning of skeletal muscle, brain and blood cells, and has a role in reproduction Protects Vitamin A and carotene from destruction by oxidation	Liver and other meat, eggs Milk Green leafy vegetables Whole grain cereals
Vitamin K	Maintains normal clotting functions of the blood	Pork liver, yolk of egg Green leafy vegetables Lettuce Cauliflower

How can I determine whether I am one of those rare people who need vitamin supplements?

If your diet includes vitamin rich foods, the chances are you're getting all you need. The most reliable means of determining vitamin deficiency is through blood analysis. It is true that certain symptoms (e.g., night blindness, bleeding gums, cracking at corners of mouth) indicate possible vitamin deficiencies, but they are only indications, not proof. A blood test is needed to confirm or deny these indications.

Why not take some vitamins to supplement my diet, just to be sure?

Even if you can afford these vitamins, supplementing your diet in this manner may not be the most desirable thing. It may set precedents that may be difficult to break. If your small children observe you pill popping they may pick up these habits through non-verbal learning.

It has been established that the best source of necessary vitamins is common table foods. It has never been proven that the vitamins taken in pills are fully absorbed into the human system. Once the tissues are saturated, much of the excess of concentrated vitamins is excreted in the body's waste products. Vitamins C and B are water soluble, and quantitites in excess of the body's needs are excreted.

There can be too much of a good thing. Vitamins A and D are fat soluble, meaning they can be stored in fat tissues and accumulated over time. Taken in larger doses than necessary, vitamins A and D can create a condition called hyper-vitaminosis–too many vitamins in the body. This condition is a mild poisoning that creates the symptoms of tiredness, anorexia, weakness, nausea, vomiting, and swelling in the lower extremities.[1]

Can vegetarians get all the nutrients they need by only eating pure vegetables?

Yes, it is possible for a vegetarian to balance his diet. But there are vegetarians and vegetarians. For some types of vegetarians, it could be extremely difficult.

The pure vegetarian eats only foods from vegetable-fruit sources. This requires the person to consume foods high in certain nutrients over and over again. Variety is highly re-stricted and there may be deficiencies in certain nutrients (protein, calcium).

The lacto-vegetarian consumes milk and milk products as well as fruits and vegetables, thereby increasing the quality of his protein intake and insuring an adequate calcium intake. Without milk products, calcium is very difficult to come by on an all-vegetable diet.

The ovo-vegetarian consumes eggs from various sources, especially chickens. Eggs are a good source of high-quality protein, phosphorus, iron, vitamins A, B-2, and D. Eggs also constitute an important source of vitamin B-12, often found to be deficient in the diets of pure and lacto-vegetarians. Inade-quate supplies of vitamin B-12, which is richly supplied in meats, can contribute to pernicious anemia.

The lacto-ovo-vegetarian consumes milk products and eggs. He is the vegetarian most likely to have a balanced diet.

The pseudovegetarian may believe he is a vegetarian, but in reality only avoids meat in the form of beef, lamb, and pork. He consumes milk, eggs, fish, seafoods, and often poultry. The pseudovegetarian can have a balanced diet, particularly if he allows himself fish and other seafood.

Many vegetarians have a missionary zeal for their practices and expound on the advantages of their diets over the typical fat-saturated American diet. They claim they feel better (probably because they are more conscious of health and nutrition); consume fewer calories (because they eat less meat, and consequently less fat); have more regular bowel movements (the fibrous tissue in vegetables aids in the elimination of solid wastes); and subsist on a much smaller food budget than their meat-consuming friends (meat is the most expensive of the Four Food Groups).

I hear a lot of talk about the hazards of food additives. Just what are food additives?

In general terms, a food additive is a very small amount of an ingredient added to a food to achieve a specific technical effect, e.g. to delay spoilage. Food additives may be classified by function: flavor enhancers, stabilizers or thickeners, leavening agents, acidity controllers, emulsifiers, preservatives, firming agents, processing aids, effervescents, curing agents, and color additives. Flavoring agents are the most widely used of the food additives. Some of the seasonings we all use every day of our lives, such as sugar and salt, are actually additives.

Who watches food additives and measures their safety?

Food additives are regulated by the Food and Drug Administration. However, the F.D.A. is inadequately staffed and has been since the early 1960s. With an ever-increasing volume of food products being released to consumers, this underfunded wing of the government should itself be fortified.

Are these food additives harmful?

Contrary to what some profit-motivated health food promoters would have you believe, food additives are "generally recognized as safe" (GRAS) by the F.D.A. Food additives are not poisonous in their recommended amounts. On the contrary, without some of these additives, particularly the preservatives, much of our food supply would spoil. Thus, some additives actually prevent certain illnesses associated with consuming perishable foods that would otherwise have undergone spoilage. As an indication of the merits of additives, it is interesting to note that most health food promoters recommend consumption of higher quantities of lecithin for the dietary control of cholesterol. Lecithin is also used as a food additive (an emulsifying agent), and is to be routinely found in most candy bars today.

Can food additives cause cancer?

The Food and Drug Administration is required by law to prohibit any additives that will cause cancer in animals, regardless of the amount used in the experiments. Because they produced tumors in experimental animals, cyclamates were removed from the market, even though a human being would have to consume more than four hundred cans of diet soda per day for an extended period of time to ingest the amount that was used in the studies. Furthermore, in the experiment the chemical was placed directly into the animal's bladder, which is not the normal physiological process.

As an example of the way this works, compare sleeping pills, which are not banned, with cyclamates, which are. Four hundred sleeping pills could kill you much more surely than four hundred cans of diet soda would. However, since sleeping pills are not known to produce cancer, the law does not prohibit them.

How many food additives have been approved by the Food and Drug Administration?

There are approximately 1830 food additives that have been approved for use. As an example of what they are and of the quantitites in which they are consumed, consider the following facts. The average female adult consumes more food additives on a yearly basis than her body weight (130 pounds, on the average). Sugar accounts for 102 of those pounds, salt for 15 pounds, corn syrup 8.4 pounds, dextrose 4.2 pounds, and approximately 1,800 other food additives account for the remaining pound.[2]

Is it possible to avoid consuming additives?

Unless you exclude sugar, salt, corn syrup, and dextrose from the category of food additives, it is almost impossible to avoid them. Check the ingredients of almost any product you normally consume and note the long list of food additives. Additives are listed in descending order by quantity. You will note that the quantities are generally very small.

In the quiz below, try to guess the food on the basis of its ingredients. The results may surprise you.

Guess the Food

In the exercise below, ten packaged food items are described by the additives they contain. The ingredients are listed in descending order of quantity, with major ingredients listed first. Guess the foods that are made up of these ingre-

dients. Check your answers against those given at the end of
the exercise.

1. Corn syrup solids, vegetable fat, sodium caseinate, di-
    potassium phosphate, emulsifier, sodium silicoaluminate,
    artificial flavor, and artificial colors.

    _____

2. Carbonated water, caramel color, flavorings, phosphoric
    acid, sodium saccharin, 1/40th of 1% sodium bensoate as a
    preservative.

    _____

3. Skim milk, sucrose, sodium caseinate, cocoa, vegetable oil,
    artificial flavor, potassium citrate, purified cellulose, cal-
    cium phosphate, sodium chloride, sodium ascorbate, car-
    boymathyl cellulose, ferric orthophosphate, artificial
    colors, calcium carrageenin, vitamin E acetate,
    niacinamides, calcium pantothenate, magnesium sulfate,
    thiamine hydrochloride, cupric sulfate, riboflavin, vi-
    tamin A, pyridoxine hydrochloride, folic acid, potassium
    iodine, vitamin D-2, vitamin B-12.

    _____

4. Sugar, citric acid, monocalcium phosphate, natural lemon
    flavor, gum arabic, lemon juice dried with corn solids,
    vitamin C, partially hydrogenated coconut oil, vitamin A,
    tricalcium phosphate, artificial color, BHA.

    _____

5. Sugar, shortening (with freshness preserver), water,
    cocoa processed with alkali, corn syrup, wheat and corn

starch, mono- and diglycerides, nonfat dry milk, salt, polysorbate 60, artificial and natural flavors, potassium sorbate, citric acid, soy lecithin, sodium phosphate, pectin, dextrose, sodium citrate.

---

6. Enriched egg noodles, salt, hydrolyzed milk and vegetable protein, dextrin, chicken fat, dehydrated chicken, natural flavorings, onion powder, MSG, yeast extract, silicon dioxide, cornstarch, potato starch, parsley, gum acacia, turmeric, hydrogenated vegetable oil, disodium inosinate, disodium guanylate.

---

7. Water, sugar, syrup, fruit juices and purees (concentrated apple, cherry, orange, and pineapple juices, papaya and guave purees, passion-fruit juice), citric acid, natural fruit flavors, vitamin C, caramel color, artificial color.

---

8. Malto-dextrins, citric acid, gum arabic, imitation flavors, salt, and artificial color.

---

9. Dehydrated vegetables (potatoes, onion, parsley, garlic), hydrolyzed vegetable protein, salt, vegetable protein, vegetable shortening, lactose, dextrins, beef extract solids, sodium caseinate, flavorings, sugar, potassium phosphate, citric acid, caramel color, monosodium glutamate, sodium sulfate, BHA.

---

10. Liver, meat by-products, soy flour, soybean, salt, caramel color, potassium chloride cellulose gum, vitamin A palmitate (stability improved) D-activated animal stero (source of Vitamin D), di-alpha tocopheryl acetate (source of vitamin E), riboflavin supplement, niacin, vitamin B-12 supplement, mendadione dimethyl pyrmidinol bisulfite (source of vitamin K activity), choline chloride, BHT (a preservative), citric acid, methionine, hydroxy analogue calcium, thiamine mononitrate, pyridoxine hydrochloride, magnesium oxide, manganous oxide, iron (ferrous sulfate), copper oxide, zinc oxide, cobalt carbonate, ethylene diamine, dihydroiodite, charcoal and water sufficient for processing.

Answers:

1. Carnation Coffee-mate Non-Dairy Creamer
2. TAB, Artificially Sweetened Dietary Carbonated Beverage
3. Slender, Diet Food for Weight Control, chocolate fudge flavor
4. Kool-Aid, Sugar-Sweetened Soft Drink Mix, imitation lemonade mix
5. Betty Crocker Ready-To-Spread Frosting, Flavored Chocolate
6. Lipton Cup-a-Soup, Chicken Noodle Soup with Chicken Meat
7. Hawaiian Punch, Cherry Royal
8. Nestle's Quik, imitation strawberry flavor
9. Betty Crocker Hamburger Helper, hash dinner
10. ALPO liver chunks and meat by-products for dogs

Is our food supply safe? Does it ever become contaminated?

People who work in food production generally avoid the foods produced at their place of employment. They may have seen, and possibly contributed to, unsanitary working conditions.

Food supplies do occasionally become contaminated. The *F.D.A. Reports*, a publication of the Food and Drug Administration that is available at most college libraries and most agricultural services, regularly releases lists of foods, specifying brand names, that have been discovered to be contaminated. The Agency imposes a cease-and-desist order withdrawing these foods from the market.

Below are some items on food contamination selected more or less at random from the *FDA Report.*

> *The Food and Drug Administration reported that Hollywood Brands have voluntarily recalled from stores and wholesalers 400,000 Hollywood Butter Nut caramel and peanut bars, and Hollywood Big Time caramel peanut nougats, after FDA inspectors found rodent hairs in some of the candy. By that time 350,000 of the 400,000 bars had been sold and presumably eaten, according to the FDA.*

Rodent hair in food suggests fecal contamination. Rodents in cleaning themselves pull out some hairs, ingest them, and expel them in their excrement.

> *The FDA announced in September that more than one-half million Oh Henry Nut Rolls had been*

recalled for possible salmonella contamination. An FDA spokesman said that the type of salmonella involved can cause intestinal infections and diarrhea.

The Food and Drug Administration reported that Affy Tapple, Inc., Coopersburg, Pa., recalled a shipment of Affy Tapple Caramel Coated Apples from Washington, D. C. area stores after a 9-year-old Alexandria, Va., child was cut on the thumb by a razor blade imbedded in one of the apples.

In August the Campbell Soup Company took the initiative of recalling all chicken-vegetable soup packed in its plant in Paris, Tex. Motive: Botulia toxin was found in cans of that soup embossed with the code number 07p13-70x and packed in that plant on July 15. The chicken-vegetable soup had been distributed in 16 states. Campbell also recalled cans of vegetarian vegetable soup packed in the Paris plant and coded 15-CT-7BIX. Campbell termed the second recall "a precautionary measure" based on the "remote possibility" of contamination by botulin toxin.

Two years ago in Delaware, a consumer found a mouse sliced up in a loaf of Bond bread. FDA inspectors traced the loaf to the Market Street, Philadelphia, bakery of Bond Baking Co. In a six-day inspection of the bakery, the FDA said it discovered extensive infestation by mice. During one day's inspection, 25 mice were spotted. Bags of flour and sesame seed were found to have been contaminated by mice.

FDA inspectors in Denver seized a shipment of chocolate mint flavored Carnation Instant Breakfast after tests showed insect filth in the breakfast food product. A court default decree ordered the shipment destroyed.

Horn and Hardart pleaded guilty to the following violations, among others: some 7700 pounds of flour and sponge-cake base contaminated with insects; 20 pounds of cake dough and 30 pounds of shelled pecans containing rodent excreta; mouse excreta, and dead insects on the bakery floor; unclean window ledges, screens, walls, ceilings, and floors, peeling paint on the cake-room ceiling; and street doors that were not rodent proof.

The Food and Drug Administration announced that the Cook Chocolate Co., of Chicago, was recalling some one million pounds of candy after an FDA analysis found samples of the candy to be contaminated with salmonella, a bacteria that can cause food poisoning. According to the FDA, most of the candy had been earmarked for fundraising sales by Boy Scouts and church groups.

The Food and Drug Administration reported that S & W Fine Foods, San Francisco, withdrew about 18,000 16-ounce jars of S & W Sweet Sour Red Cabbage from wholesale and retail channels after receiving numerous complaints from purchasers who said they found glass particles in the jars. Nearly 50,000 jars of the suspect cabbage, packed by Aunt Nellies Food, Inc., Clyman, Wis., had already been sold by the time the others were taken off the market.

Sunshine Biscuit Co., Dayton, Ohio, withdrew 103,000 cases of shredded wheat, cookies, sweet goods, and iced products from the market, according to the Food and Drug Administration, after samples were found to be contaminated with ronnel, a pesticide. The amount of the suspect food bought by consumers is unknown. It was sold under the brand names Sunshine, Fame, Staff and Marsh.

Pepsi-Cola Buffalo Bottling Co., Cheektowaga, N. Y., recalled an undetermined amount of Pepsi-Cola, Teem, Diet Pepsi and Hires Root Beer after an inspection by the Food and Drug Administration revealed mold contamination in some containers of the beverages. The sodas, which were packaged in uncoded bottles, were distributed in various areas of New York State. Earlier this year, Coca-Cola Bottling Co., of New York, Inc., Tonawanda, N.Y., recalled its products on two separate occasions, following the discovery by the FDA of mold contamination.

Reports such as these can give us a lot of help in sticking to diet! If you're wondering how you can avoid contamination in foods, perhaps you have concluded that you should avoid canned and packaged foodstuffs and use as much as possible fresh provisions. At least the impurities, if any, will be your own.

What role does advertising play in the food industry?

The truth behind the trite statement, "It pays to advertise," is especially evident in relation to the food industry as witnessed by the number of unnecessary products that are successfully promoted. Advertising is very expensive and the cost is passed on to the consumer through increased prices. A one-minute commercial on prime time television costs the promoter about $60,000 every time the commercial is aired.

Advertisers are not in business to tell the truth; they are in business to promote products and to proliferate profits. Many advertisements are packed with half-truths, conveyed either by direct statement or by innuendo. They prey on the ignorance and gullibility of the consumer.

For example, their commercials state that Carnation Instant Breakfast mixed with milk will provide as much mineral value as two strips of bacon, as much energy value as two slices of toast, as much vitamin value as a glass of orange juice, and as much protein value as an egg. This information is true, but very misleading—especially when pictorially presented. The bacon, toast, orange juice, and egg are depicted inside a glass of Instant Breakfast mixed with milk, implying that all the nutritional benefits of those foods are provided by Carnation Instant Breakfast. *Truth:* As claimed, only the mineral of the bacon, only the protein of the egg, only the vitamins of the orange juice will be derived. As left unstated, the other nutrients normally found in these foods are not supplied by Carnation Instant Breakfast. *Further truth:* If the Carnation Instant Breakfast were mixed with water, it would provide very few nutrients. In fact, by itself, this breakfast powder is little more than flavoring with certain vitamins added. The majority of the nutrients mentioned in the advertisement are supplied by the *milk*. The chief value of the product would seem to be to make milk more palatable.

Madison Avenue cooks up clever advertising schemes to create a need for the product being pushed. It's sad to realize that many indigent families' cupboards are void of nutritious foodstuffs but stocked with many dollars' worth of food supplements and vitamins.

Recommended for further reading is Vance Packard's classic book, *The Hidden Persuaders*[3]. Even though the specifics in this book are dated, it will arouse a healthy skepticism about all advertisements and perhaps lead you to re-evaluate your shopping practices.

Advertising consultant Nicholas Samstag might have been speaking for all his colleagues in advertising when he wrote in the *Saturday Review of Literature* in 1966:

> *Every member of the advertising establishment spends most of his working hours concocting half-truths and then trying to distribute them as widely and persuasively as possible. This is his job. He is not paid to tell the whole truth or even to know it. Usually he isn't told it. When he comes across facts that weaken or fail to strengthen his case, he automatically ignores them, buries or eliminates them, not only from his thinking but from his consciousness as well. By working hard at this assignment (and it isn't an easy one), he gradually succeeds at it. And so he forgets where the truth is, masters his half-truths, and his income begins to climb.*

Now, let it be clearly understood that I see nothing wrong about this from the point of view of advertising . . . .

REFERENCES

1. Consumer's Union, "Multiple Vitamin Supplements," (Chapter 14 in:) *The Medicine Show,* (Revised edition), Mount Vernon, New York: Consumer's Union, 1970, pp. 97-98.

2. Hall, Richard L., "Food Additives," *Nutrition Today,* July-August, 1973, pp. 20-28.

3. Packard, Vance, *The Hidden Persuaders,* New York: Pocket Books, 1958.

Looking Back;
Looking Forward

The real beginning of your weight control program will take place after you finish this book. Triumph in thinning from within begins when you make up your mind to try it. Action-based behavior is what burns calories. Thinking won't do it.

In this book you have been given opportunities to explore your own feelings and to acquire information about sensible nutrition and reasonable diet plans. You have also been encouraged to *act* on these values. Your progress so far is the first step of a long walk. Just as when you were a toddler, you practiced walking until it became an unconscious pattern, so must you make a determined, conscious effort to count calories and take advantage of movement opportunities until such value-based behavior becomes a pattern of your life.

Diet Diary

If you've been responding in writing to the strategies throughout this book, by now you've accumulated an extensive diary of thoughts and commitments. Look back over what you wrote weeks and even months ago. You just might be surprised. Have you lived up to your commitments? goals? predictions?

At this point in your program, are there areas in which you've changed your opinions?

Have you established new activity or diet patterns?

Are you more conscious of portion size? Calorie content?

Are you aware of the balance between intake and outgo? Can you look at a piece of fruit and think, "That banana will cost me a 17-minute walk"?

Are you less likely to purchase or consume products because of their appealing packages?

Do you eat more slowly?

Have you acquired enough knowledge to rationally analyze fad diets?

Do you semiconsciously follow the Four Food Groups or some other nutritionally sound alternative?

When you catch yourself falling prey to food cues (eating just because it's there) do you stop long enough to ask, "Do I really *need* this?"

Unused knowledge keeps no better than raw fish. Weight won't come off because you've read a book on weight control. *Thin From Within* is an action-based book. People can reach you and teach you, but in the final analysis only *you* can do something about it. You are the only one who can make a difference in your life.

Appendix A

Bibliography: What to Read; What Not to Read*

The following books are reliable sources of weight control information:

1. Berland, Theodore, *Rating the Diets*. Skokie, Illinois: Consumer Guide, 1974.

   > An excellent and revealing analysis of everything you need to know about diets. It reveals the truth about specific diets and exposes the myths and mysteries of popular weight control schemes. Mr. Berland's exposé is extraordinarily thorough. The best book currently available. Well documented.

2. Danowski, T.S., M.D. *Sustained Weight Control—The Individual Approach*. F.A. Davis Co., Philadelphia, 1969.

   Reviewed by Committee on Nutrition, American Heart Association.

   > "Written in layman's language, this book emphasizes that motivation and reorganization of eating

---

* This recommended list and the following list of unreliable books was compiled in part from "Selected Nutrition References," Massachusetts Department of Public Health, Nutrition Program, Boston, Massachusetts: January, 1972.

300

patterns are the keys to permanent weight loss. The roles of genetic patterns and emotional factors in obesity are discussed."

3. Glenn, Morton, M.D. *How to Get Thinner Once and For All.* E.P. Dutton Co., New York, 1965.

A sensible, valuable guide based on sound nutrition for those seriously concerned with a weight problem. Dr. Glenn discusses the roles of life styles, motivation, and portion control in weight loss and maintenance.

4. Joliffe, Norman, M.D. *Reduce And Stay Reduced On The Prudent Diet.* Simon and Schuster, New York, 1964.

Reviewed by Ohio Department of Health.

"Reports of a seven-year study on men in New York City who adhered to a regime called the Prudent Diet."

5. Kain, Ida J. and Mildred Gibson. *Stay Slim For Life.* Doubleday and Co., Inc., Garden City, New York, revised, 1967.

Reviewed by Washington State Department of Health.

"Subtitled 'Diet Cookbook for Overweight Millions', this popular yet scientific explanation of weight and attractive and practical menus and recipes can be recommended without reservation."

6. Levine, M.I. and J.H. Seligmann, *Your Overweight Child.* New York: The World Publishing Company, 1970.

7. Mayer, Jean. *Overweight: Causes, Cost, and Control.* En-

glewood Cliffs, N. J.: Prentice-Hall, Inc., 1968.

> A world authority on weight control, Dr. Mayer of Harvard University discusses the multifaceted nature of overweight and the implications of the research.

8. Stuart, R.B. and B. Davis. *Slim Chance in a Fat World: Behavioral Control of Obesity.* Research Press Company, 1972.

> An excellent approach to the solution of obesity through behavior modification. Stresses the role of activity in conjunction with diet. A well-documented book.

9. Wyden, Peter, et al. *The All-In-One Diet Annual.* Bantam Book Co., New York, 1970.

> A complete guide to weight reduction based on sound nutritional principles for dieting. Mr. Wyden expects the reader to choose a diet plan that fits his life style. The caloric values of common foods are given so they can be adapted to your own lo-cal plan.

10. Wyden, Peter. *The Overweight Society.* William Morrow and Co., New York, 1965.

> A well-written commentary on the attitude of society today toward the problem of obesity and overweight. Details and evaluations are given of the fad diets and popular reducing diets. The author advocates dieting under the direction of a physician, and keeping weight down by a permanent change in eating habits as well as through some type of exercise.

11. Wyden, Peter and Barbara. *How the Doctors Diet.* New York: Trident Press, 1968.

> An analysis of the diets of 89 top medical authorities and their families reveals exactly what they eat and how they exercise to get thin. After compiling the results, general guidelines are suggested which reveal that doctors *do* practice what they preach.

The following books are not recommended as reliable sources of information about nutrition and weight-control.

1. Abrahamson, E.M. and A.W. Pezet. *Body, Mind and Sugar.* New York: Holt, Rinehart and Winston, Inc., 1965.

2. Anchell, M. *How I Lost 36,000 Pounds.* Detroit: Harlo Press, 1964.

3. Atkins, Robert C. *Dr. Atkins' Diet Revolution.* New York: Bantam Books, Inc., 1972.

4. Davis, Adelle. *Let's Eat Right to Keep Fit.* New York: Harcourt Brace, 1954.

5. Davis, Adelle. *Let's Get Well.* A Practical Guide to Renewed Health Through Nutrition. New York: Harcourt, Brace and World, Inc., 1965.

6. Davis, Adelle. *Let's Have Healthy Children.* New York: Harcourt Brace. 1959.

7. Fredericks, C. and H. Bailey, *Good Facts and Fallacies:*

The Intelligent Person's Guide to Nutrition and Health. New York: The Julian Press, 1965.

8. Fredericks, C. *The Carlton Fredericks Cookbook for Good Nutrition.* Philadelphia: J.B. Lippincott Co., 1960.

9. Fredericks, C. *Dr. Carlton Fredericks' Low-Carbohydrate Diet.* New York: 1964 (New Printing).

10. Hauser, G. *The New Diet Does It.* New York: G.P. Putnam's Sons, 1960.

11. Jarvis, D.C. *Arthritis and Folk Medicine.* Greenwich, Conn.: Fawcett Publications, Inc., (Crest Book) 1962.

12. Jarvis, D.C. *Folk Medicine—A Vermont Doctor's Guide to Good Health.* New York: Holt, Rinehart and Winston, Inc., 1958.

13. Pauling, Linus. *Vitamin C and The Common Cold.* San Francisco: Witt, Freeman and Co., 1970.

14. Rodale, J.I. and Staff. *Our Poisoned Earth and Sky.* Emmaus, Pennsylvania: Rodale Press Inc., 1964.

15. Rodale, J.I. and Staff. *The Organic Directory.* Emmaus, Pennsylvania: Rodale Press, 1971.

16. Stillman, I.M. and S.S. Baker. *The Doctor's Quick Weight Loss Diet.* New York: Dell Publishing Co., Inc., 1968.

17. Stillman, I.M. and S.S. Baker. *Doctor's Inches Off Diet.* New York: Dell, 1970.

18. Stillman, I.M. and S.S. Baker. *Doctor's Quick Teenage Diet.* New York: Paperback Library, 1972.

19. Taller, H. *Calories Don't Count.* New York: Simon and Schuster, 1961.

20. West, Ruth. *Stop Dieting! Start Losing!* New York: Bantam Books, 1957.

21. West, Ruth. *The Teenage Diet Book.* New York: Bantam Books, 1958. (revised, 1970).

Appendix B

Sample Diet Models

I generally avoid recommending specific diet plans for the following reasons:

1. Most diets are too restrictive. They are too full of do's and don'ts.

2. Most diets are too monotonous; therefore, the drop-out rate is high.

3. Most diets rely too heavily on certain foods, such as fish, for example. If you don't happen to like these foods, you are not offered many alternatives.

4. Most diets are not well balanced nutritionally.

5. Most diets fail to teach the dieter how to achieve his own caloric regulation. Many plans don't even mention calories. For a diet to work, the caloric principle must be understood by the dieter and he must be willing and knowledgeable enough to exercise self-regulation.

You can develop your own diet based on your own tastes and preferences. Your diet should be balanced and you should reduce your daily caloric intake by no more than 800 calories.

No food need be completely eliminated from your diet; you need only to reduce the amount to keep it within sane caloric limits. The sample diet models below are based on the four food groups and suggest limits within each group. The diet models do not list specific food items. You do the choosing within each group. If you follow the caloric suggestions within each food group you will fulfill the 2:2:4:4 daily suggested servings. With this balanced diet approach, YOU select the foods YOU prefer within the suggested caloric limitations. In this way the five pitfalls listed above are avoided.

Three model plans are suggested here - 1200, 1600, and 2000 calorie diets. Select the plan that best fits your needs. Each model is based on three well-balanced meals per day so that fatigue due to dietary deficiencies (so common on fad diets) will not be experienced. You can also be assured that you are receiving all of the necessary nutrients in just about their proper amounts. Expensive vitamin and mineral supplementation then becomes unnecessary.

Careful selection of snacks can add nutrient fortification to the four food group foundation. Nutritious snacks are limited only by your imagination. In general, teenagers would be wise to select snacks from the milk group; women in their childbearing years from sources rich in iron; teenage women from both.

Whichever of these diet models you may choose to follow, increased activity should be a regular part of your plan. Activity will not only burn up calories while toning up muscles, but it will also increase your resting metabolic rate for up to 24 hours. Furthermore, activity will actually regulate your appetite.

1200 CALORIE FOOD INTAKE PLAN

CAUTION: This plan is not recommended for everyone. A

1200 calorie plan is recommended only for persons who are small in stature (under 5' 3"), or physically (medically) unable to increase their activity levels. If you have not realized your desired weight loss on the 1600 calorie plan, you may decide to try the 1200 calorie plan.

Too limited a calorie intake may cause irritability. To restrict calorie intake to less than 1200 may disturb the body's homeostasis, or natural balance. Further restriction of calories (especially by elimination of a food group) would jeopardize the nutritional adequacy of your diet plan.

BREAKFAST - 280 calories:

Bread & Cereal Group	=	60 calories
Fruit & Vegetable Group (C)	=	70 "
(½) Milk Group	=	50 "
(½) Meat Group	=	100 "

LUNCH - 430 calories:

(2) Bread & Cereal Group	=	120 calories
Fruit & Vegetable Group	=	50 "
Milk Group	=	90 "
Meat Group	=	170 "

DINNER - 490 calories:

Bread & Cereal Group	=	60 calories
(2) Fruit & Vegetable Group (A)	=	90 "
Milk Group	=	90 "
Meat Group	=	250 "

Snacks - Extremely low items such as celery sticks, gum, low-calorie soft drinks.

Activity Plan:

1. Minimize your use of labor (calorie) saving devices.

2. Walk at a moderate pace (3 m.p.h.) for 20-30 minutes daily over and above your pre-plan levels.

3. Do moderate toning activities (such as those on T.V. exercise programs) at least twice per week.

4. At least twice per week engage in some activity that will cause you to be out of breath for at least 30 seconds. (Example: Walking up several flights of stairs or climbing uphill.)

1600 CALORIE FOOD INTAKE PLAN

This 1600 calorie plan is the most popular. It provides adequate nutrients and a palatable but prudent use of calories. When combined with the activity recommendations, this plan promotes a steady fat weight loss. Most sedentary business persons, homemakers, and some teenagers find it quite agreeable to pursue this plan during prolonged battles of the bulge. Do not eliminate any servings from the recommended food groups.

BREAKFAST - 320 calories:

Bread & Cereal Group   = 100 calories
Fruit & Vegetable Group (C) = 70   "
(½) Milk Group   = 50   "
(½) Meat Group   = 100   "

LUNCH - 555 calories:

(2) Bread & Cereal Group   = 170 calories
Fruit & Vegetable Group   = 80   "
Milk Group   = 95   "
Meat Group   = 210   "

DINNER - 625 calories:

Bread & Cereal Group   = 90 calories
(2) Fruit & Vegetable Group (A) = 125   "
Milk Group   = 120   "
Meat Group   = 290   "

SNACKS - 100 calories:

Snack calories can be used, within stated limits, for any-thing you desire or crave. However, the prudent person selects sensible snacks from the four food groups (such as raisins, nuts, yogurt, etc.) to further fortify his reduced calorie food plan. Teenagers should select their snacks from the milk group.

Activity Plan:

1. Minimize your use of labor (calorie) saving devices.

2. Walk moderately (3 m.p.h.) for 20-30 minutes

daily over and above your pre-plan level.

3. Do moderate toning activities (such as those on T.V. exercise programs) at least twice per week.

4. At least twice per week engage in some activity that will cause you to be out of breath for at least 30 seconds. (Example: Walking up several flights of stairs or uphill.)

2000 CALORIE FOOD INTAKE PLAN

This plan is recommended for active or tall women (above 5' 5"), active teenagers, and most non-sedentary males. Some persons may not experience a one-to-two pound weekly weight loss on this plan. If not, switch to the 1600 calorie plan, or make a 200-250 calorie reduction without eliminating any of the suggested groups. You can, however, eliminate the snack of 150 calories.

BREAKFAST - 455 calories:

Bread and Cereal Group	= 125	calories
Fruit and Vegetable Group (C)	= 85	"
(½) Milk Group	= 95	"
(½) Meat Group	= 150	"

LUNCH - 655 calories:

(2) Bread & Cereal Group	= 175	calories
Fruit & Vegetable Group	= 90	"
Milk Group	= 140	"
Meat Group	= 250	"

DINNER - 740 calories:

Bread & Cereal Group   = 100 calories
(2) Fruit & Vegetable Group (A) = 130   ”
Milk Group   = 165   ”
Meat Group   = 345   ”

SNACKS - 150 calories:

Snack calories can be used, within stated limits, for anything you desire or crave. However, the prudent person selects sensible snacks from the four food groups (such as raisins, nuts, yogurt, etc.) to further fortify his reduced food plan. Teenagers should select their snacks from the milk group.

Activity Plan:

1. Minimize your use of labor (calorie) saving devices.

2. Walk moderately (3 m.p.h) for 20 minutes twice daily, or for 40 minutes once daily over and above your pre-plan level.

3. Do moderate toning activities (such as those on T.V. exercise programs) at least two or three times per week.

4. At least twice per week engage in some activity that will cause you to be out of breath for about a minute. (Example: Walking up several flights of stairs or uphill.)

Appendix C

Nutritive Value of Foods

TABLE 1.—NUTRITIVE VALUES OF

[Dashes in the columns for nutrients show that no suitable value could be found although

	Food, approximate measure, and weight (in grams)		Water	Food energy	Pro-tein	Fat
	MILK, CHEESE, CREAM, IMITATION CREAM; RELATED PRODUCTS					
		Grams	*Per-cent*	*Calo-ries*	*Grams*	*Grams*
	Milk:					
	Fluid:					
1	Whole, 3.5% fat_____ 1 cup_____	244	87	160	9	9
2	Nonfat (skim)_____ 1 cup_____	245	90	90	9	Trace
3	Partly skimmed, 2% 1 cup_____ nonfat milk solids added.	246	87	145	10	5
	Canned, concentrated, undiluted:					
4	Evaporated, un- 1 cup_____ sweetened.	252	74	345	18	20
5	Condensed, sweet- 1 cup_____ ened.	306	27	980	25	27
	Dry, nonfat instant:					
6	Low-density (1⅓ 1 cup_____ cups needed for re-constitution to 1 qt.).	68	4	245	24	Trace
7	High-density (⅞ cup 1 cup_____ needed for recon-stitution to 1 qt.).	104	4	375	37	1
	Buttermilk:					
8	Fluid, cultured, made 1 cup_____ from skim milk.	245	90	90	9	Trace
9	Dried, packaged_____ 1 cup_____	120	3	465	41	6
	Cheese:					
	Natural:					
	Blue or Roquefort type:					
10	Ounce_____ 1 oz._____	28	40	105	6	9
11	Cubic inch_____ 1 cu. in._____	17	40	65	4	5

THE EDIBLE PART OF FOODS

there is reason to believe that a measurable amount of the nutrient may be present]

Fatty acids			Carbo-hy-drate	Cal-cium	Iron	Vita-min A value	Thia-min	Ribo-flavin	Niacin	Ascor-bic acid
Satu-rated (total)	Unsaturated									
	Oleic	Lin-oleic								
Grams	*Grams*	*Grams*	*Grams*	*Milli-grams*	*Milli-grams*	*Inter-national units*	*Milli-grams*	*Milli-grams*	*Milli-grams*	*Milli-grams*
5	3	Trace	12	288	0.1	350	0.07	0.41	0.2	2
-----	-----	-----	12	296	.1	10	.09	.44	.2	2
3	2	Trace	15	352	.1	200	.10	.52	.2	2
11	7	1	24	635	.3	810	.10	.86	.5	3
15	9	1	166	802	.3	1,100	.24	1.16	.6	3
-----	-----	-----	35	879	.4	[1]20	.24	1.21	.6	5
-----	-----	-----	54	1,345	.6	[1]30	.36	1.85	.9	7
-----	-----	-----	12	296	.1	10	.10	.44	.2	2
3	2	Trace	60	1,498	.7	260	.31	2.06	1.1	------
5	3	Trace	1	89	.1	350	.01	.17	.3	0
3	2	Trace	Trace	54	.1	210	.01	.11	.2	0

TABLE 1.—NUTRITIVE VALUES OF

[Dashes in the columns for nutrients show that no suitable value could be found although

	Food, approximate measure, and weight (in grams)		Water	Food energy	Pro-tein	Fat
	MILK, CHEESE, CREAM, IMITATION CREAM; RELATED PRODUCTS—Con.		*Per-cent*	*Calo-ries*	*Grams*	*Grams*
		Grams				
12	Camembert, pack-aged in 4-oz. pkg. with 3 wedges per pkg.	1 wedge_____ 38	52	115	7	9
	Cheddar:					
13	Ounce_____	1 oz._____ 28	37	115	7	9
14	Cubic inch_____	1 cu. in._____ 17	37	70	4	6
	Cottage, large or small curd:					
	Creamed:					
15	Package of 12-oz., net wt.	1 pkg._____ 340	78	360	46	14
16	Cup, curd pressed down.	1 cup_____ 245	78	260	33	10
	Uncreamed:					
17	Package of 12-oz., net wt.	1 pkg._____ 340	79	290	58	1
18	Cup, curd pressed down.	1 cup_____ 200	79	170	34	1
	Cream:					
19	Package of 8-oz., net wt.	1 pkg._____ 227	51	850	18	86
20	Package of 3-oz., net wt.	1 pkg._____ 85	51	320	7	32
21	Cubic inch_____	1 cu. in._____ 16	51	60	1	6
	Parmesan, grated:					
22	Cup, pressed down_	1 cup_____ 140	17	655	60	43
23	Tablespoon_____	1 tbsp._____ 5	17	25	2	2
24	Ounce_____	1 oz._____ 28	17	130	12	9
	Swiss:					
25	Ounce_____	1 oz._____ 28	39	105	8	8
26	Cubic inch_____	1 cu. in._____ 15	39	55	4	4

THE EDIBLE PART OF FOODS—Continued

there is reason to believe that a measurable amount of the nutrient may be present]

Fatty acids			Carbo-hy-drate	Cal-cium	Iron	Vita-min A value	Thia-min	Ribo-flavin	Niacin	Ascor-bic acid
Satu-rated (total)	Unsaturated									
	Oleic	Lin-oleic								
Grams	*Grams*	*Grams*	*Grams*	*Milli-grams*	*Milli-grams*	*Inter-national units*	*Milli-grams*	*Milli-grams*	*Milli-grams*	*Milli-grams*
5	3	Trace	1	40	0.2	380	0.02	0.29	0.3	0
5	3	Trace	1	213	.3	370	.01	.13	Trace	0
3	2	Trace	Trace	129	.2	230	.01	.08	Trace	0
8	5	Trace	10	320	1.0	580	.10	.85	.3	0
6	3	Trace	7	230	.7	420	.07	.61	.2	0
1	Trace	Trace	9	306	1.4	30	.10	.95	.3	0
Trace	Trace	Trace	5	180	.8	20	.06	.56	.2	0
48	28	3	5	141	.5	3,500	.05	.54	.2	0
18	11	1	2	53	.2	1,310	.02	.20	.1	0
3	2	Trace	Trace	10	Trace	250	Trace	.04	Trace	0
24	14	1	5	1,893	.7	1,760	.03	1.22	.3	0
1	Trace	Trace	Trace	68	Trace	60	Trace	.04	Trace	0
5	3	Trace	1	383	.1	360	.01	.25	.1	0
4	3	Trace	1	262	.3	320	Trace	.11	Trace	0
2	1	Trace	Trace	139	.1	170	Trace	.06	Trace	0

TABLE 1.—NUTRITIVE VALUES OF

[Dashes in the columns for nutrients show that no suitable value could be found although

	Food, approximate measure, and weight (in grams)	Water	Food energy	Pro-tein	Fat
	MILK, CHEESE, CREAM, IMITATION CREAM; RELATED PRODUCTS—Con.	*Per-cent*	*Calo-ries*	*Grams*	*Grams*
	Grams				
	Pasteurized processed cheese:				
	American:				
27	Ounce............ 1 oz.......... 28	40	105	7	9
28	Cubic inch........ 1 cu. in...... 18	40	65	4	5
	Swiss:				
29	Ounce............ 1 oz.......... 28	40	100	8	8
30	Cubic inch........ 1 cu. in...... 18	40	65	5	5
	Pasteurized process cheese food, American:				
31	Tablespoon......... 1 tbsp....... 14	43	45	3	3
32	Cubic inch.......... 1 cu. in...... 18	43	60	4	4
33	Pasteurized process 1 oz.......... 28 cheese spread, American.	49	80	5	6
	Cream:				
34	Half-and-half (cream 1 cup........ 242 and milk).	80	325	8	28
35	1 tbsp....... 15	80	20	1	2
36	Light, coffee or table... 1 cup........ 240	72	505	7	49
37	1 tbsp....... 15	72	30	1	3
38	Sour................ 1 cup........ 230	72	485	7	47
39	1 tbsp....... 12	72	25	Trace	2
40	Whipped topping 1 cup........ 60 (pressurized).	62	155	2	14
41	1 tbsp....... 3	62	10	Trace	1
	Whipping, unwhipped (volume about double when whipped):				
42	Light.............. 1 cup........ 239	62	715	6	75
43	1 tbsp....... 15	62	45	Trace	5
44	Heavy............. 1 cup........ 238	57	840	5	90
45	1 tbsp....... 15	57	55	Trace	6

THE EDIBLE PART OF FOODS—Continued

there is reason to believe that a measurable amount of the nutrient may be present]

Fatty acids			Carbo-hy-drate	Cal-cium	Iron	Vita-min A value	Thia-min	Ribo-flavin	Niacin	Ascor-bic acid
Satu-rated (total)	Unsaturated									
	Oleic	Lin-oleic								
Grams	*Grams*	*Grams*	*Grams*	*Milli-grams*	*Milli-grams*	*Inter-national units*	*Milli-grams*	*Milli-grams*	*Milli-grams*	*Milli-grams*
5	3	Trace	1	198	.3	350	.01	.12	Trace	0
3	2	Trace	Trace	122	.2	210	Trace	.07	Trace	0
4	3	Trace	1	251	.3	310	Trace	.11	Trace	0
3	2	Trace	Trace	159	.2	200	Trace	.07	Trace	0
2	1	Trace	1	80	.1	140	Trace	.08	Trace	0
2	1	Trace	1	100	.1	170	Trace	.10	Trace	0
3	2	Trace	2	160	.2	250	Trace	.15	Trace	0
15	9	1	11	261	.1	1,160	.07	.39	.1	2
1	1	Trace	1	16	Trace	70	Trace	.02	Trace	Trace
27	16	1	10	245	.1	2,020	.07	.36	.1	2
2	1	Trace	1	15	Trace	130	Trace	.02	Trace	Trace
26	16	1	10	235	.1	1,930	.07	.35	.1	2
1	1	Trace	1	12	Trace	100	Trace	.02	Trace	Trace
8	5	Trace	6	67	------	570	------	.04	------	------
Trace	Trace	Trace	Trace	3	------	30	------	Trace	------	------
41	25	2	9	203	.1	3,060	.05	.29	.1	2
3	2	Trace	1	13	Trace	190	Trace	.02	Trace	Trace
50	30	3	7	179	.1	3,670	.05	.26	.1	2
3	2	Trace	1	11	Trace	230	Trace	.02	Trace	Trace

TABLE 1.—NUTRITIVE VALUES OF

[Dashes in the columns for nutrients show that no suitable value could be found although

	Food, approximate measure, and weight (in grams)			Water	Food energy	Pro- tein	Fat
	MILK, CHEESE, CREAM, IMITATION CREAM; RELATED PRODUCTS						
			Grams	*Per- cent*	*Calo- ries*	*Grams*	*Grams*
	Imitation cream products (made with vege- table fat):						
	Creamers:						
46	Powdered_____	1 cup_____	94	2	505	4	33
47		1 tsp._____	2	2	10	Trace	1
48	Liquid (frozen)_____	1 cup_____	245	77	345	3	27
49		1 tbsp._____	15	77	20	Trace	2
50	Sour dressing (imita- tion sour cream) made with nonfat dry milk.	1 cup_____	235	72	440	9	38
51		1 tbsp._____	12	72	20	Trace	2
	Whipped topping:						
52	Pressurized_____	1 cup_____	70	61	190	1	17
53		1 tbsp._____	4	61	10	Trace	1
54	Frozen_____	1 cup_____	75	52	230	1	20
55		1 tbsp._____	4	52	10	Trace	1
56	Powdered, made with whole milk.	1 cup_____	75	58	175	3	12
57		1 tbsp._____	4	58	10	Trace	1
	Milk beverages:						
58	Cocoa, homemade_____	1 cup_____	250	79	245	10	12
59	Chocolate-flavored drink made with skim milk and 2% added butterfat.	1 cup_____	250	83	190	8	6
	Malted milk:						
60	Dry powder, approx. 3 heaping tea- spoons per ounce.	1 oz._____	28	3	115	4	2
61	Beverage_____	1 cup_____	235	78	245	11	10

THE EDIBLE PART OF FOODS—Continued

there is reason to believe that a measurable amount of the nutrient may be present]

Fatty acids			Carbo-hy-drate	Cal-cium	Iron	Vita-min A value	Thia-min	Ribo-flavin	Niacin	Ascor-bic acid
Satu-rated (total)	Unsaturated									
	Oleic	Lin-oleic								
Grams	*Grams*	*Grams*	*Grams*	*Milli-grams*	*Milli-grams*	*Inter-national units*	*Milli-grams*	*Milli-grams*	*Milli-grams*	*Milli-grams*
31	1	0	52	21	.6	[2] 200	------	------	Trace	------
Trace	Trace	0	1	1	Trace	[2] Trace	------	------	------	------
25	1	0	25	29	------	[2] 100	0	0	------	------
1	Trace	0	2	2	------	[2] 10	0	0	------	------
35	1	Trace	17	277	.1	10	.07	.38	.2	1
2	Trace	Trace	1	14	Trace	Trace	Trace	Trace	Trace	Trace
15	1	0	9	5	------	[2] 340	------	0	------	------
1	Trace	0	Trace	Trace	------	[2] 20	------	0	------	------
18	Trace	0	15	5	------	[2] 560	------	0	------	------
1	Trace	0	1	Trace	------	[2] 30	------	0	------	------
10	1	Trace	15	62	Trace	[2] 330	.02	.08	.1	Trace
1	Trace	Trace	1	3	Trace	[2] 20	Trace	Trace	Trace	Trace
7	4	Trace	27	295	1.0	400	.10	.45	.5	3
3	2	Trace	27	270	.5	210	.10	.40	.3	3
------	------	------	20	82	.6	290	.09	.15	.1	0
------	------	------	28	317	.7	590	.14	.49	.2	2

TABLE 1.—NUTRITIVE VALUES OF

[Dashes in the columns for nutrients show that no suitable value could be found although

	Food, approximate measure, and weight (in grams)	Water	Food energy	Pro-tein	Fat
	MILK, CHEESE, CREAM, IMITATION CREAM; RELATED PRODUCTS				
		Per-cent	*Calo-ries*	*Grams*	*Grams*
	Milk desserts:				
62	Custard, baked_____ 1 cup_____ 265	77	305	14	15
	Ice cream:				
63	Regular (approx. ½ gal._____1,064	63	2,055	48	113
	10% fat).				
64	1 cup_____ 133	63	255	6	14
65	3 fl. oz. cup__ 50	63	95	2	5
66	Rich (approx. 16% ½ gal._____1,188	63	2,635	31	191
	fat).				
67	1 cup_____ 148	63	330	4	24
	Ice milk:				
68	Hardened_____ ½ gal._____1,048	67	1,595	50	53
69	1 cup_____ 131	67	200	6	7
70	Soft-serve_____ 1 cup_____ 175	67	265	8	9
	Yoghurt:				
71	Made from partially 1 cup_____ 245	89	125	8	4
	skimmed milk.				
72	Made from whole milk_ 1 cup_____ 245	88	150	7	8
	EGGS				
	Eggs, large, 24 ounces per dozen:				
	Raw or cooked in shell or with nothing added:				
73	Whole, without shell_ 1 egg_____ 50	74	80	6	6
74	White of egg_____ 1 white_____ 33	88	15	4	Trace
75	Yolk of egg_____ 1 yolk_____ 17	51	60	3	5
76	Scrambled with milk 1 egg_____ 64	72	110	7	8
	and fat.				

THE EDIBLE PART OF FOODS—Continued

there is reason to believe that a measurable amount of the nutrient may be present]

Fatty acids			Carbo-hy-drate	Cal-cium	Iron	Vita-min A value	Thia-min	Ribo-flavin	Niacin	Ascor-bic acid
Satu-rated (total)	Unsaturated									
	Oleic	Lin-oleic								
Grams	*Grams*	*Grams*	*Grams*	*Milli-grams*	*Milli-grams*	*Inter-national units*	*Milli-grams*	*Milli-grams*	*Milli-grams*	*Milli-grams*
7	5	1	29	297	1.1	930	.11	.50	.3	1
62	37	3	221	1,553	.5	4,680	.43	2.23	1.1	11
8	5	Trace	28	194	.1	590	.05	.28	.1	1
3	2	Trace	10	73	Trace	220	.02	.11	.1	1
105	63	6	214	927	.2	7,840	.24	1.31	1.2	12
13	8	1	27	115	Trace	980	.03	.16	.1	1
29	17	2	235	1,635	1.0	2,200	.52	2.31	1.0	10
4	2	Trace	29	204	.1	280	.07	.29	.1	1
5	3	Trace	39	273	.2	370	.09	.39	.2	2
2	1	Trace	13	294	.1	170	.10	.44	.2	2
5	3	Trace	12	272	.1	340	.07	.39	.2	2
2	3	Trace	Trace	27	1.1	590	.05	.15	Trace	0
			Trace	3	Trace	0	Trace	.09	Trace	0
2	2	Trace	Trace	24	.9	580	.04	.07	Trace	0
3	3	Trace	1	51	1.1	690	.05	.18	Trace	0

TABLE 1.—NUTRITIVE VALUES OF

[Dashes in the columns for nutrients show that no suitable value could be found although

	Food, approximate measure, and weight (in grams)	Water	Food energy	Pro- tein	Fat
	MEAT, POULTRY, FISH, SHELLFISH; RELATED PRODUCTS				
		Grams	*Per- cent*	*Calo- ries*	*Grams*	*Grams*
77	Bacon, (20 slices per lb. 2 slices_____ raw), broiled or fried, crisp.	15	8	90	5	8
	Beef,[3] cooked:					
	Cuts braised, simmered, or pot-roasted:					
78	Lean and fat_____ 3 ounces_____	85	53	245	23	16
79	Lean only_____ 2.5 ounces___	72	62	140	22	5
	Hamburger (ground beef), broiled:					
80	Lean_____ 3 ounces_____	85	60	185	23	10
81	Regular_____ 3 ounces_____	85	54	245	21	17
	Roast, oven-cooked, no liquid added:					
	Relatively fat, such as rib:					
82	Lean and fat_____ 3 ounces_____	85	40	375	17	34
83	Lean only_____ 1.8 ounces___	51	57	125	14	7
	Relatively lean, such as heel of round:					
84	Lean and fat_____ 3 ounces_____	85	62	165	25	7
85	Lean only_____ 2.7 ounces___	78	65	125	24	3
	Steak, broiled:					
	Relatively, fat, such as sirloin:					
86	Lean and fat_____ 3 ounces_____	85	44	330	20	27
87	Lean only_____ 2.0 ounces___	56	59	115	18	4
	Relatively, lean, such as round:					
88	Lean and fat_____ 3 ounces_____	85	55	220	24	13
89	Lean only_____ 2.4 ounces___	68	61	130	21	4
	Beef, canned:					
90	Corned beef_____ 3 ounces_____	85	59	185	22	10
91	Corned beef hash_____ 3 ounces_____	85	67	155	7	10
92	Beef, dried or chipped____ 2 ounces_____	57	48	115	19	4
93	Beef and vegetable stew__ 1 cup_____	235	82	210	15	10
94	Beef potpie, baked, 4¼- 1 pie_____ inch diam., weight before baking about 8 ounces.	227	55	560	23	33

THE EDIBLE PART OF FOODS—Continued

there is reason to believe that a measurable amount of the nutrient may be present]

Fatty acids			Carbo-hy-drate	Cal-cium	Iron	Vita-min A value	Thia-min	Ribo-flavin	Niacin	Ascor-bic acid
Satu-rated (total)	Unsaturated									
	Oleic	Lin-oleic								
Grams	*Grams*	*Grams*	*Grams*	*Milli-grams*	*Milli-grams*	*Inter-national units*	*Milli-grams*	*Milli-grams*	*Milli-grams*	*Milli-grams*
3	4	1	1	2	.5	0	.08	.05	.8	------
8	7	Trace	0	10	2.9	30	.04	.18	3.5	------
2	2	Trace	0	10	2.7	10	.04	.16	3.3	------
5	4	Trace	0	10	3.0	20	.08	.20	5.1	------
8	8	Trace	0	9	2.7	30	.07	.18	4.6	------
16	15	1	0	8	2.2	70	.05	.13	3.1	------
3	3	Trace	0	6	1.8	10	.04	.11	2.6	------
3	3	Trace	0	11	3.2	10	.06	.19	4.5	------
1	1	Trace	0	10	3.0	Trace	.06	.18	4.3	------
13	12	1	0	9	2.5	50	.05	.16	4.0	------
2	2	Trace	0	7	2.2	10	.05	.14	3.6	------
6	6	Trace	0	10	3.0	20	.07	.19	4.8	------
2	2	Trace	0	9	2.5	10	.06	.16	4.1	------
5	4	Trace	0	17	3.7	20	.01	.20	2.9	------
5	4	Trace	9	11	1.7	------	.01	.08	1.8	------
2	2	Trace	0	11	2.9	------	.04	.18	2.2	------
5	4	Trace	15	28	2.8	2,310	.13	.17	4.4	15
9	20	2	43	32	4.1	1,860	0.25	0.27	4.5	7

TABLE 1.—NUTRITIVE VALUES OF

[Dashes in the columns for nutrients show that no suitable value could be found although

	Food, approximate measure, and weight (in grams)			Water	Food energy	Pro-tein	Fat
	MEAT, POULTRY, FISH, SHELLFISH; RELATED PRODUCTS—Continued						
	Chicken, cooked:		*Grams*	*Per-cent*	*Calo-ries*	*Grams*	*Grams*
95	Flesh only, broiled_____	3 ounces_____	85	71	115	20	3
	Breast, fried, ½ breast:						
96	With bone_____	3.3 ounces___	94	58	155	25	5
97	Flesh and skin only__	2.7 ounces___	76	58	155	25	5
	Drumstick, fried:						
98	With bone_____	2.1 ounces___	59	55	90	12	4
99	Flesh and skin only__	1.3 ounces___	38	55	90	12	4
100	Chicken, canned, boneless	3 ounces___	85	65	170	18	10
101	Chicken potpie, baked 4¼-inch diam., weight before baking about 8 ounces.	1 pie_____	227	57	535	23	31
	Chili con carne, canned:						
102	With beans_____	1 cup_____	250	72	335	19	15
103	Without beans_____	1 cup_____	255	67	510	26	38
104	Heart, beef, lean, braised_	3 ounces_____	85	61	160	27	5
	Lamb,[3] cooked:						
105	Chop, thick, with bone, broiled.	1 chop, 4.8 ounces.	137	47	400	25	33
106	Lean and fat_____	4.0 ounces___	112	47	400	25	33
107	Lean only_____	2.6 ounces___	74	62	140	21	6
	Leg, roasted:						
108	Lean and fat_____	3 ounces_____	85	54	235	22	16
109	Lean only_____	2.5 ounces___	71	62	130	20	5
	Shoulder, roasted:						
110	Lean and fat_____	3 ounces_____	85	50	285	18	23
111	Lean only_____	2.3 ounces___	64	61	130	17	6

THE EDIBLE PART OF FOODS—Continued

there is reason to believe that a measurable amount of the nutrient may be present]

Fatty acids			Carbo-hy-drate	Cal-cium	Iron	Vita-min A value	Thia-min	Ribo-flavin	Niacin	Ascor-bic acid
Satu-rated (total)	Unsaturated									
	Oleic	Lin-oleic								
Grams	*Grams*	*Grams*	*Grams*	*Milli-grams*	*Milli-grams*	*Inter-national units*	*Milli-grams*	*Milli-grams*	*Milli-grams*	*Milli-grams*
1	1	1	0	8	1.4	80	.05	.16	7.4	------
1	2	1	1	9	1.3	70	.04	.17	11.2	------
1	2	1	1	9	1.3	70	.04	.17	11.2	------
1	2	1	Trace	6	.9	50	.03	.15	2.7	------
1	2	1	Trace	6	.9	50	.03	.15	2.7	------
3	4	2	0	18	1.3	200	.03	.11	3.7	3
10	15	3	42	68	3.0	3,020	.25	.26	4.1	5
7	7	Trace	30	80	4.2	150	.08	.18	3.2	------
18	17	1	15	97	3.6	380	.05	.31	5.6	------
------	------	------	1	5	5.0	20	.21	1.04	6.5	1
18	12	1	0	10	1.5	-------	.14	.25	5.6	------
18	12	1	0	10	1.5	-------	.14	.25	5.6	------
3	2	Trace	0	9	1.5	-------	.11	.20	4.5	------
9	6	Trace	0	9	1.4	-------	.13	.23	4.7	------
3	2	Trace	0	9	1.4	-------	.12	.21	4.4	------
13	8	1	0	˙9	1.0	-------	.11	.20	4.0	------
3	2	Trace	0	8	1.0	-------	.10	.18	3.7	------

TABLE 1.—NUTRITIVE VALUES OF

Dashes in the columns for nutrients show that no suitable value could be found although

	Food, approximate measure, and weight (in grams)		Water	Food energy	Pro- tein	Fat
	MEAT, POULTRY, FISH, SHELLFISH; RELATED PRODUCTS—Continued		*Per- cent*	*Calo- ries*	*Grams*	*Grams*
		Grams				
112	Liver, beef, fried_____ 2 ounces_____	57	57	130	15	6
	Pork, cured, cooked:					
113	Ham, light cure, lean 3 ounces_____ and fat, roasted.	85	54	245	18	19
	Luncheon meat:					
114	Boiled ham, sliced___ 2 ounces_____	57	59	135	11	10
115	Canned, spiced or 2 ounces_____ unspiced.	57	55	165	8	14
	Pork, fresh,[3] cooked:					
116	Chop, thick, with bone_ 1 chop, 3.5 ounces.	98	42	260	16	21
117	Lean and fat_____ 2.3 ounces___	66	42	260	16	21
118	Lean only_____ 1.7 ounces___	48	53	130	15	7
	Roast, oven-cooked, no liquid added:					
119	Lean and fat_____ 3 ounces_____	85	46	310	21	24
120	Lean only_____ 2.4 ounces___	68	55	175	20	10
	Cuts, simmered:					
121	Lean and fat_____ 3 ounces_____	85	46	320	20	26
122	Lean only_____ 2.2 ounces___	63	60	135	18	6
	Sausage:					
123	Bologna, slice, 3-in. 2 slices_____ diam. by ⅛ inch.	26	56	80	3	7
124	Braunschweiger, slice 2 slices_____ 2-in. diam. by ¼ inch.	20	53	65	3	5
125	Deviled ham, canned___ 1 tbsp._____	13	51	45	2	4
126	Frankfurter, heated 1 frank_____ (8 per lb. purchased pkg.).	56	57	170	7	15
127	Pork links, cooked 2 links_____ (16 links per lb. raw).	26	35	125	5	11
128	Salami, dry type_____ 1 oz._____	28	30	130	7	11

THE EDIBLE PART OF FOODS—Continued

there is reason to believe that a measurable amount of the nutrient may be present]

Fatty acids			Carbo-hy-drate	Cal-cium	Iron	Vita-min A value	Thia-min	Ribo-flavin	Niacin	Ascor-bic acid
Satu-rated (total)	Unsaturated									
	Oleic	Lin-oleic								
Grams	Grams	Grams	Grams	Milli-grams	Milli-grams	Inter-national units	Milli-grams	Milli-grams	Milli-grams	Milli-grams
------	------	------	3	6	5.0	30,280	.15	2.37	9.4	15
7	8	2	0	8	2.2	0	.40	.16	3.1	------
4	4	1	0	6	1.6	0	.25	.09	1.5	------
5	6	1	1	5	1.2	0	.18	.12	1.6	------
8	9	2	0	8	2.2	0	.63	.18	3.8	------
8	9	2	0	8	2.2	0	.63	.18	3.8	------
2	3	1	0	7	1.9	0	.54	.16	3.3	------
9	10	2	0	9	2.7	0	.78	.22	4.7	------
3	4	1	0	9	2.6	0	.73	.21	4.4	------
9	11	2	0	8	2.5	0	.46	.21	4.1	------
2	3	1	0	8	2.3	0	.42	.19	3.7	------
------	------	------	Trace	2	.5	-------	.04	.06	.7	------
------	------	------	Trace	2	1.2	1,310	.03	.29	1.6	------
2	2	Trace	0	1	.3	-------	.02	.01	.2	------
------	------	------	1	3	.8	-------	.08	.11	1.4	------
4	5	1	Trace	2	.6	0	.21	.09	1.0	------
------	------	------	Trace	4	1.0	-------	.10	.07	1.5	------

TABLE 1.—NUTRITIVE VALUES OF

[Dashes in the columns for nutrients show that no suitable value could be found although

	Food, approximate measure, and weight (in grams)			Water	Food energy	Pro-tein	Fat
			Grams	Per-cent	Calo-ries	Grams	Grams

MEAT, POULTRY, FISH, SHELLFISH; RELATED PRODUCTS—Continued

Fish and shellfish—Continued

	Food, approximate measure, and weight		Grams	Per-cent	Calo-ries	Grams	Grams
129	Salami, cooked_____ 1 oz._____		28	51	90	5	7
130	Vienna, canned (7 sausages per 5-oz. can).	1 sausage____	16	63	40	2	3
	Veal, medium fat, cooked, bone removed:						
131	Cutlet_____ 3 oz._____		85	60	185	23	9
132	Roast_____ 3 oz._____		85	55	230	23	14
	Fish and shellfish:						
133	Bluefish, baked with table fat.	3 oz._____	85	68	135	22	4
	Clams:						
134	Raw, meat only_____ 3 oz._____		85	82	65	11	1
135	Canned, solids and liquid.	3 oz._____	85	86	45	7	1
136	Crabmeat, canned_____ 3 oz._____		85	77	85	15	2
137	Fish sticks, breaded, cooked, frozen; stick 3¾ by 1 by ½ inch.	10 sticks or 8 oz. pkg.	227	66	400	38	20
138	Haddock, breaded, fried 3 oz._____		85	66	140	17	5
139	Ocean perch, breaded, fried.	3 oz._____	85	59	195	16	11
140	Oysters, raw, meat only (13–19 med. selects).	1 cup_____	240	85	160	20	4
141	Salmon, pink, canned__ 3 oz._____		85	71	120	17	5
142	Sardines, Atlantic, canned in oil, drained solids.	3 oz._____	85	62	175	20	9
143	Shad, baked with table fat and bacon.	3 oz._____	85	64	170	20	10

THE EDIBLE PART OF FOODS—Continued

there is reason to believe that a measurable amount of the nutrient may be present]

Fatty acids			Carbo-hy-drate	Cal-cium	Iron	Vita-min A value	Thia-min	Ribo-flavin	Niacin	Ascor-bic acid
Satu-rated (total)	Unsaturated									
	Oleic	Lin-oleic								
Grams	*Grams*	*Grams*	*Grams*	*Milli-grams*	*Milli-grams*	*Inter-national units*	*Milli-grams*	*Milli-grams*	*Milli-grams*	*Milli-grams*
------	------	------	Trace	3	.7	-------	.07	.07	1.2	------
------	------	------	Trace	1	.3	-------	.01	.02	.4	------
5	4	Trace	------	9	2.7	-------	.06	.21	4.6	------
7	6	Trace	0	10	2.9	-------	.11	.26	6.6	------
------	------	------	0	25	.6	40	.09	.08	1.6	------
------	------	------	2	59	5.2	90	.08	.15	1.1	8
------	------	------	2	47	3.5	-------	.01	.09	.9	------
------	------	------	1	38	.7	-------	.07	.07	1.6	------
5	4	10	15	25	0.9	-------	0.09	0.16	3.6	------
1	3	Trace	5	34	1.0	-------	.03	.06	2.7	2
------	------	------	6	28	1.1	-------	.08	.09	1.5	------
------	------	------	8	226	13.2	740	.33	.43	6.0	------
1	1	Trace	0	4 167	.7	60	.03	.16	6.8	------
------	------	------	0	372	2.5	190	.02	.17	4.6	------
------	------	------	0	20	.5	20	.11	.22	7.3	------

TABLE 1.—NUTRITIVE VALUES OF

[Dashes in the columns for nutrients show that no suitable value could be found although

	Food, approximate measure, and weight (in grams)		Water	Food energy	Pro-tein	Fat
	MEAT, POULTRY, FISH, SHELLFISH; RELATED PRODUCTS—Continued					
	Fish and shellfish—Continued	*Grams*	*Per-cent*	*Calo-ries*	*Grams*	*Grams*
144	Shrimp, canned, meat__ 3 oz._____	85	70	100	21	1
145	Swordfish, broiled 3 oz._____ with butter or margarine.	85	65	150	24	5
146	Tuna, canned in oil, 3 oz._____ drained solids.	85	61	170	24	7
	MATURE DRY BEANS AND PEAS, NUTS, PEANUTS; RELATED PRODUCTS					
147	Almonds, shelled, whole 1 cup_____ kernels.	142	5	850	26	77
	Beans, dry:					
	Common varieties as Great Northern, navy, and others:					
	Cooked, drained:					
148	Great Northern___ 1 cup_____	180	69	210	14	1
149	Navy (pea)_____ 1 cup_____	190	69	225	15	1
	Canned, solids and liquid:					
	White with—					
150	Frankfurters 1 cup_____ (sliced).	255	71	365	19	18
151	Pork and 1 cup_____ tomato sauce.	255	71	310	16	7
152	Pork and sweet 1 cup_____ sauce.	255	66	385	16	12
153	Red kidney_____ 1 cup_____	255	76	230	15	1
154	Lima, cooked, 1 cup_____ drained.	190	64	260	16	1
155	Cashew nuts, roasted____ 1 cup_____	140	5	785	24	64

THE EDIBLE PART OF FOODS—Continued

there is reason to believe that a measurable amount of the nutrient may be present1

Fatty acids			Carbo-hydrate	Cal-cium	Iron	Vita-min A value	Thia-min	Ribo-flavin	Niacin	Ascor-bic acid
Satu-rated (total)	Unsaturated									
	Oleic	Lin-oleic								
Grams	*Grams*	*Grams*	*Grams*	*Milli-grams*	*Milli-grams*	*Inter-national units*	*Milli-grams*	*Milli-grams*	*Milli-grams*	*Milli-grams*
------	------	------	1	98	2.6	50	.01	.03	1.5	------
------	------	------	0	23	1.1	1,750	.03	.04	9.3	------
2	1	1	0	7	1.6	70	.04	.10	10.1	------
6	52	15	28	332	6.7	0	.34	1.31	5.0	Trace
------	------	------	38	90	4.9	0	.25	.13	1.3	0
------	------	------	40	95	5.1	0	.27	.13	1.3	0
------	------	------	32	94	4.8	330	.18	.15	3.3	Trace
2	3	1	49	138	4.6	330	.20	.08	1.5	5
4	5	1	54	161	5.9	-------	.15	.10	1.3	------
------	------	------	42	74	4.6	10	.13	.10	1.5	------
------	------	------	49	55	5.9	-------	.25	.11	1.3	------
11	45	4	41	53	5.3	140	.60	.35	2.5	------

TABLE 1.—NUTRITIVE VALUES OF

Dashes in the columns for nutrients show that no suitable value could be found although

	Food, approximate measure, and weight (in grams)			Water	Food energy	Protein	Fat
	MATURE DRY BEANS AND PEAS, NUTS, PEANUTS; RELATED PRODUCTS—Con.		*Grams*	*Percent*	*Calories*	*Grams*	*Grams*
	Coconut, fresh, meat only:						
156	Pieces, approx. 2 by 2 by ½ inch.	1 piece_____	45	51	155	2	16
157	Shredded or grated, firmly packed.	1 cup_____	130	51	450	5	46
158	Cowpeas or blackeye peas, dry, cooked.	1 cup_____	248	80	190	13	1
159	Peanuts, roasted, salted, halves.	1 cup_____	144	2	840	37	72
160	Peanut butter_____	1 tbsp._____	16	2	95	4	8
161	Peas, split, dry, cooked___	1 cup_____	250	70	290	20	1
162	Pecans, halves_____	1 cup_____	108	3	740	10	77
163	Walnuts, black or native, chopped.	1 cup_____	126	3	790	26	75
	VEGETABLES AND VEGETABLE PRODUCTS						
	Asparagus, green:						
	Cooked, drained:						
164	Spears, ½-in. diam. at base.	4 spears_____	60	94	10	1	Trace
165	Pieces, 1½ to 2-in. lengths.	1 cup_____	145	94	30	3	Trace
166	Canned, solids and liquid.	1 cup_____	244	94	45	5	1
	Beans:						
167	Lima, immature seeds, cooked, drained.	1 cup_____	170	71	190	13	1

THE EDIBLE PART OF FOODS—Continued

there is reason to believe that a measurable amount of the nutrient may be present]

Fatty acids			Carbo-hy-drate	Cal-cium	Iron	Vita-min A value	Thia-min	Ribo-flavin	Niacin	Ascor-bic acid
Satu-rated (total)	Unsaturated									
	Oleic	Lin-oleic								
Grams	*Grams*	*Grams*	*Grams*	*Milli-grams*	*Milli-grams*	*Inter-national units*	*Milli-grams*	*Milli-grams*	*Milli-grams*	*Milli-grams*
14	1	Trace	4	6	.8	0	.02	.01	.2	1
39	3	Trace	12	17	2.2	0	.07	.03	.7	4
-----	-----	-----	34	42	3.2	20	.41	.11	1.1	Trace
16	31	21	27	107	3.0	-------	.46	.19	24.7	0
2	4	2	3	9	.3	-------	.02	.02	2.4	0
-----	-----	-----	52	28	4.2	100	.37	.22	2.2	-----
5	48	15	16	79	2.6	140	.93	.14	1.0	2
4	26	36	19	Trace	7.6	380	.28	.14	.9	-----
-----	-----	-----	2	13	.4	540	.10	.11	.8	16
-----	-----	-----	5	30	.9	1,310	.23	.26	2.0	38
-----	-----	-----	7	44	4.1	1,240	.15	.22	2.0	37
-----	-----	-----	34	80	4.3	480	.31	.17	2.2	29

TABLE 1.—NUTRITIVE VALUES OF

[Dashes in the columns for nutrients show that no suitable value could be found although

Food, approximate measure, and weight (in grams)			Water	Food energy	Pro- tein	Fat
VEGETABLES AND VEGETABLE PRODUCTS—Continued		Grams	Per- cent	Calo- ries	Grams	Grams
Snap:						
Green:						
168	Cooked, drained___ 1 cup_____	125	92	30	2	Trace
169	Canned, solids 1 cup_____ and liquid.	239	94	45	2	Trace
	Yellow or wax:					
170	Cooked, drained___ 1 cup_____	125	93	30	2	Trace
171	Canned, solids 1 cup_____ and liquid.	239	94	45	2	1
172	Sprouted mung beans, 1 cup_____ cooked, drained.	125	91	35	4	Trace
	Beets:					
	Cooked, drained, peeled:					
173	Whole beets, 2-in. 2 beets_____ diam.	100	91	30	1	Trace
174	Diced or sliced_____ 1 cup_____	170	91	55	2	Trace
175	Canned, solids and 1 cup_____ liquid.	246	90	85	2	Trace
176	Beet greens, leaves and 1 cup_____ stems, cooked, drained.	145	94	25	3	Trace
	Blackeye peas. See Cowpeas.					
	Broccoli, cooked, drained:					
177	Whole stalks, 1 stalk_____ medium size.	180	91	45	6	1
178	Stalks cut into ½-in. 1 cup_____ pieces.	155	91	40	5	1
179	Chopped, yield from 1⅜ cups____ 10-oz. frozen pkg.	250	92	65	7	1

THE EDIBLE PART OF FOODS—Continued

there is reason to believe that a measurable amount of the nutrient may be present]

Fatty acids			Carbo-hydrate	Cal-cium	Iron	Vita-min A value	Thia-min	Ribo-flavin	Niacin	Ascor-bic acid
Satu-rated (total)	Unsaturated									
	Oleic	Lin-oleic								
Grams	*Grams*	*Grams*	*Grams*	*Milli-grams*	*Milli-grams*	*Inter-national units*	*Milli-grams*	*Milli-grams*	*Milli-grams*	*Milli-grams*
-----	-----	-----	7	63	.8	680	.09	.11	.6	15
-----	-----	-----	10	81	2.9	690	.07	.10	.7	10
-----	-----	-----	6	63	0.8	290	0.09	0.11	0.6	16
-----	-----	-----	10	81	2.9	140	.07	.10	.7	12
-----	-----	-----	7	21	1.1	30	.11	.13	.9	8
-----	-----	-----	7	14	.5	20	.03	.04	.3	6
-----	-----	-----	12	24	.9	30	.05	.07	.5	10
-----	-----	-----	19	34	1.5	20	.02	.05	.2	7
-----	-----	-----	5	144	2.8	7,400	.10	.22	.4	22
-----	-----	-----	8	158	1.4	4,500	.16	.36	1.4	162
-----	-----	-----	7	136	1.2	3,880	.14	.31	1.2	140
-----	-----	-----	12	135	1.8	6,500	.15	.30	1.3	143

TABLE 1.—NUTRITIVE VALUES OF

[Dashes in the columns for nutrients show that no suitable value could be found although

	Food, approximate measure, and weight (in grams)			Water	Food energy	Pro-tein	Fat
	VEGETABLES AND VEGETABLE PRODUCTS—Continued		*Grams*	*Per-cent*	*Calo-ries*	*Grams*	*Grams*
180	Brussels sprouts, 7–8 sprouts (1¼ to 1½ in. diam.) per cup, cooked.	1 cup_____	155	88	55	7	1
	Cabbage:						
	Common varieties:						
	Raw:						
181	Coarsely shredded or sliced.	1 cup_____	70	92	15	1	Trace
182	Finely shredded or chopped.	1 cup_____	90	92	20	1	Trace
183	Cooked_____	1 cup_____	145	94	30	2	Trace
184	Red, raw, coarsely shredded.	1 cup_____	70	90	20	1	Trace
185	Savoy, raw, coarsely shredded.	1 cup_____	70	92	15	2	Trace
186	Cabbage, celery or Chinese, raw, cut in 1-in. pieces.	1 cup_____	75	95	10	1	Trace
187	Cabbage, spoon (or pakchoy), cooked.	1 cup_____	170	95	25	2	Trace
	Carrots:						
	Raw:						
188	Whole, 5½ by 1 inch, (25 thin strips).	1 carrot_____	50	88	20	1	Trace
189	Grated_____	1 cup_____	110	88	45	1	Trace
190	Cooked, diced_____	1 cup_____	145	91	45	1	Trace
191	Canned, strained or chopped (baby food).	1 ounce_____	28	92	10	Trace	Trace
192	Cauliflower, cooked, flowerbuds.	1 cup_____	120	93	25	3	Trace

THE EDIBLE PART OF FOODS—Continued

there is reason to believe that a measurable amount of the nutrient may be present]

Fatty acids			Carbo-hy-drate	Cal-cium	Iron	Vita-min A value	Thia-min	Ribo-flavin	Niacin	Ascor-bic acid
Satu-rated (total)	Unsaturated									
	Oleic	Lin-oleic								
Grams	*Grams*	*Grams*	*Grams*	*Milli-grams*	*Milli-grams*	*Inter-national units*	*Milli-grams*	*Milli-grams*	*Milli-grams*	*Milli-grams*
------	------	------	10	50	1.7	810	.12	.22	1.2	135
------	------	------	4	34	.3	90	.04	.04	.2	33
------	------	------	5	44	.4	120	.05	.05	.3	42
------	------	------	6	64	.4	190	.06	.06	.4	48
------	------	------	5	29	.6	30	.06	.04	.3	43
------	------	------	3	47	.6	140	.04	.06	.2	39
------	------	------	2	32	.5	110	.04	.03	.5	19
------	------	------	4	252	1.0	5,270	.07	.14	1.2	26
------	------	------	5	18	.4	5,500	.03	.03	.3	4
------	------	------	11	41	.8	12,100	.06	.06	.7	9
------	------	------	10	48	.9	15,220	.08	.07	.7	9
------	------	------	2	7	.1	3,690	.01	.01	.1	1
------	------	------	5	25	.8	70	.11	.10	.7	66

TABLE 1.—NUTRITIVE VALUES OF

[Dashes in the columns for nutrients show that no suitable value could be found although

	Food, approximate measure, and weight (in grams)			Water	Food energy	Pro-tein	Fat
			Grams	Per-cent	Calo-ries	Grams	Grams
	VEGETABLES AND VEGETABLE PRODUCTS—Continued						
	Celery, raw:						
193	Stalk, large outer, 8 by about 1½ inches, at root end.	1 stalk_____	40	94	5	Trace	Trace
194	Pieces, diced_____	1 cup_____	100	94	15	1	Trace
195	Collards, cooked_____	1 cup_____	190	91	55	5	1
	Corn, sweet:						
196	Cooked, ear 5 by 1¾ inches.[5]	1 ear_____	140	74	70	3	1
197	Canned, solids and liquid.	1 cup_____	256	81	170	5	2
198	Cowpeas, cooked, im-mature seeds.	1 cup_____	160	72	175	13	1
	Cucumbers, 10-ounce; 7½ by about 2 inches:						
199	Raw, pared_____	1 cucumber__	207	96	30	1	Trace
200	Raw, pared, center slice ⅛-inch thick.	6 slices_____	50	96	5	Trace	Trace
201	Dandelion greens, cooked_	1 cup_____	180	90	60	4	1
202	Endive, curly (includ-ing escarole).	2 ounces_____	57	93	10	1	Trace
203	Kale, leaves including stems, cooked.	1 cup_____	110	91	30	4	1
	Lettuce, raw:						
204	Butterhead, as Boston types; head, 4-inch diameter.	1 head_____	220	95	30	3	Trace
205	Crisphead, as Iceberg; head, 4¾-inch diameter.	1 head_____	454	96	60	4	Trace

THE EDIBLE PART OF FOODS—Continued

there is reason to believe that a measurable amount of the nutrient may be present]

Fatty acids			Carbo-hy-drate	Cal-cium	Iron	Vita-min A value	Thia-min	Ribo-flavin	Niacin	Ascor-bic acid
Satu-rated (total)	Unsaturated									
	Oleic	Lin-oleic								
Grams	*Grams*	*Grams*	*Grams*	*Milli-grams*	*Milli-grams*	*Inter-national units*	*Milli-grams*	*Milli-grams*	*Milli-grams*	*Milli-grams*
------	------	------	2	16	.1	100	.01	.01	.1	4
------	------	------	4	39	.3	240	.03	.03	.3	9
------	------	------	9	289	1.1	10,260	.27	.37	2.4	87
------	------	------	16	2	.5	[6] 310	.09	.08	1.0	7
------	------	------	40	10	1.0	[6] 690	.07	.12	2.3	13
------	------	------	29	38	3.4	560	.49	.18	2.3	28
------	------	------	7	35	.6	Trace	.07	.09	.4	23
------	------	------	2	8	.2	Trace	.02	.02	.1	6
------	------	------	12	252	3.2	21,060	.24	.29	------	32
------	------	------	2	46	1.0	1,870	0.04	0.08	0.3	6
------	------	------	4	147	1.3	8,140	------	------	------	68
------	------	------	6	77	4.4	2,130	.14	.13	.6	18
------	------	------	13	91	2.3	1,500	.29	.27	1.3	29

TABLE 1.—NUTRITIVE VALUES OF

[Dashes in the columns for nutrients show that no suitable value could be found although

	Food, approximate measure, and weight (in grams)		Water	Food energy	Protein	Fat
			Per-cent	Calo-ries	Grams	Grams
	VEGETABLES AND VEGETABLE PRODUCTS—Continued					
		Grams				
206	Looseleaf, or bunching varieties, leaves.	2 large_____ 50	94	10	1	Trace
207	Mushrooms, canned, solids and liquid.	1 cup_____ 244	93	40	5	Trace
208	Mustard greens, cooked__	1 cup_____ 140	93	35	3	1
209	Okra, cooked, pod 3 by ⅝ inch.	8 pods_____ 85	91	25	2	Trace
	Onions:					
	Mature:					
210	Raw, onion 2½-inch diameter.	1 onion_____ 110	89	40	2	Trace
211	Cooked_____	1 cup_____ 210	92	60	3	Trace
212	Young green, small, without tops.	6 onions_____ 50	88	20	1	Trace
213	Parsley, raw, chopped____	1 tablespoon_ 4	85	Trace	Trace	Trace
214	Parsnips, cooked_____	1 cup_____ 155	82	100	2	1
	Peas, green:					
215	Cooked_____	1 cup_____ 160	82	115	9	1
216	Canned, solids and liquid.	1 cup_____ 249	83	165	9	1
217	Canned, strained (baby food).	1 ounce_____ 28	86	15	1	Trace
218	Peppers, hot, red, without seeds, dried (ground chili powder, added seasonings).	1 tablespoon_ 15	8	50	2	2
	Peppers, sweet:					
	Raw, about 5 per pound:					
219	Green pod without stem and seeds.	1 pod_____ 74	93	15	1	Trace

THE EDIBLE PART OF FOODS—Continued

there is reason to believe that a measurable amount of the nutrient may be present]

| Satu-rated (total) | Unsaturated | | Carbo-hy-drate | Cal-cium | Iron | Vita-min A value | Thia-min | Ribo-flavin | Niacin | Ascor-bic acid |
	Oleic	Lin-oleic								
Grams	*Grams*	*Grams*	*Grams*	*Milli-grams*	*Milli-grams*	*Inter-national units*	*Milli-grams*	*Milli-grams*	*Milli-grams*	*Milli-grams*
------	------	------	2	34	.7	950	.03	.04	.2	9
------	------	------	6	15	1.2	Trace	.04	.60	4.8	4
------	------	------	6	193	2.5	8,120	.11	.19	.9	68
------	------	------	5	78	.4	420	.11	.15	.8	17
------	------	------	10	30	.6	40	.04	.04	.2	11
------	------	------	14	50	.8	80	.06	.06	.4	14
------	------	------	5	20	.3	Trace	.02	.02	.2	12
------	------	------	Trace	8	.2	340	Trace	.01	Trace	7
------	------	------	23	70	.9	50	.11	.12	.2	16
------	------	------	19	37	2.9	860	.44	.17	3.7	33
------	------	------	31	50	4.2	1,120	.23	.13	2.2	22
------	------	------	3	3	.4	140	.02	.02	.4	3
------	------	------	8	40	2.3	9,750	.03	.17	1.3	2
------	------	------	4	7	.5	310	.06	.06	.4	94

Fatty acids

TABLE 1.—NUTRITIVE VALUES OF

[Dashes in the columns for nutrients show that no suitable value could be found although

	Food, approximate measure, and weight (in grams)		Water	Food energy	Pro-tein	Fat
	VEGETABLES AND VEGETABLE PRODUCTS—Continued					
		Grams	*Per-cent*	*Calo-ries*	*Grams*	*Grams*
220	Cooked, boiled, drained 1 pod_____	73	95	15	1	Trace
	Potatoes, medium (about 3 per pound raw):					
221	Baked, peeled after baking. 1 potato_____	99	75	90	3	Trace
	Boiled:					
222	Peeled after boiling__ 1 potato_____	136	80	105	3	Trace
223	Peeled before boiling_ 1 potato_____	122	83	80	2	Trace
	French-fried, piece 2 by ½ by ½ inch:					
224	Cooked in deep fat___ 10 pieces____	57	45	155	2	7
225	Frozen, heated_____ 10 pieces____	57	53	125	2	5
	Mashed:					
226	Milk added_____ 1 cup_____	195	83	125	4	1
227	Milk and butter added. 1 cup_____	195	80	185	4	8
228	Potato chips, medium, 2-inch diameter. 10 chips_____	20	2	115	1	8
229	Pumpkin, canned_____ 1 cup_____	228	90	75	2	1
230	Radishes, raw, small, without tops. 4 radishes___	40	94	5	Trace	Trace
231	Sauerkraut, canned, solids and liquid. 1 cup_____	235	93	45	2	Trace
	Spinach:					
232	Cooked_____ 1 cup_____	180	92	40	5	1
233	Canned, drained solids_ 1 cup_____	180	91	45	5	1
	Squash:					
	Cooked:					
234	Summer, diced_____ 1 cup_____	210	96	30	2	Trace
235	Winter, baked, mashed. 1 cup_____	205	81	130	4	1

THE EDIBLE PART OF FOODS—Continued

there is reason to believe that a measurable amount of the nutrient may be present]

Fatty acids			Carbo-hy-drate	Cal-cium	Iron	Vita-min A value	Thia-min	Ribo-flavin	Niacin	Ascor-bic acid
Satu-rated (total)	Unsaturated									
	Oleic	Lin-oleic								
Grams	*Grams*	*Grams*	*Grams*	*Milli-grams*	*Milli-grams*	*Inter-national units*	*Milli-grams*	*Milli-grams*	*Milli-grams*	*Milli-grams*
------	------	------	3	7	.4	310	.05	.05	.4	70
------	------	------	21	9	.7	Trace	.10	.04	1.7	20
------	------	------	23	10	.8	Trace	.13	.05	2.0	22
------	------	------	18	7	.6	Trace	.11	.04	1.4	20
2	2	4	20	9	.7	Trace	.07	.04	1.8	12
1	1	2	19	5	1.0	Trace	.08	.01	1.5	12
------	------	------	25	47	.8	50	.16	.10	2.0	19
4	3	Trace	24	47	.8	330	.16	.10	1.9	18
2	2	4	10	8	.4	Trace	.04	.01	1.0	3
------	------	------	18	57	.9	14,590	.07	.12	1.3	12
------	------	------	1	12	.4	Trace	.01	.01	.1	10
------	------	------	9	85	1.2	120	.07	.09	.4	33
------	------	------	6	167	4.0	14,580	.13	.25	1.0	50
------	------	------	6	212	4.7	14,400	.03	.21	.6	24
------	------	------	7	52	.8	820	.10	.16	1.6	21
------	------	------	32	57	1.6	8,610	.10	.27	1.4	27

TABLE 1.—NUTRITIVE VALUES OF

[Dashes in the columns for nutrients show that no suitable value could be found although

	Food, approximate measure, and weight (in grams)			Water	Food energy	Pro-tein	Fat
			Grams	*Per-cent*	*Calo-ries*	*Grams*	*Grams*
	VEGETABLES AND VEGETABLE PRODUCTS—Continued						
	Sweetpotatoes:						
	Cooked, medium, 5 by 2 inches, weight raw about 6 ounces:						
236	Baked, peeled after baking.	1 sweet-potato.	110	64	155	2	1
237	Boiled, peeled after boiling.	1 sweet-potato.	147	71	170	2	1
238	Candied, 3½ by 2¼ inches.	1 sweet-potato.	175	60	295	2	6
239	Canned, vacuum or solid pack.	1 cup_____	218	72	235	4	Trace
	Tomatoes:						
240	Raw, approx. 3-in. diam. 2⅛ in. high; wt., 7 oz.	1 tomato____	200	94	40	2	Trace
241	Canned, solids and liquid.	1 cup_____	241	94	50	2	1
	Tomato catsup:						
242	Cup_____	1 cup_____	273	69	290	6	1
243	Tablespoon_____	1 tbsp._____	15	69	15	Trace	Trace
	Tomato juice, canned:						
244	Cup_____	1 cup_____	243	94	45	2	Trace
245	Glass (6 fl. oz.)_____	1 glass_____	182	94	35	2	Trace
246	Turnips, cooked, diced____	1 cup_____	155	94	35	1	Trace
247	Turnip greens, cooked____	1 cup_____	145	94	30	3	Trace
	FRUITS AND FRUIT PRODUCTS						
248	Apples, raw (about 3 per lb.).[5]	1 apple_____	150	85	70	Trace	Trace

THE EDIBLE PART OF FOODS—Continued

there is reason to believe that a measurable amount of the nutrient may be present]

Saturated (total)	Unsaturated Oleic	Unsaturated Linoleic	Carbohydrate	Calcium	Iron	Vitamin A value	Thiamin	Riboflavin	Niacin	Ascorbic acid
Grams	*Grams*	*Grams*	*Grams*	*Milligrams*	*Milligrams*	*International units*	*Milligrams*	*Milligrams*	*Milligrams*	*Milligrams*
-----	-----	-----	36	44	1.0	8,910	.10	.07	.7	24
-----	-----	-----	39	47	1.0	11,610	.13	.09	.9	25
2	3	1	60	65	1.6	11,030	0.10	0.08	0.8	17
-----	-----	-----	54	54	1.7	17,000	.10	.10	1.4	30
-----	-----	-----	9	24	.9	1,640	.11	.07	1.3	[7] 42
-----	-----	-----	10	14	1.2	2,170	.12	.07	1.7	41
-----	-----	-----	69	60	2.2	3,820	.25	.19	4.4	41
-----	-----	-----	4	3	.1	210	.01	.01	.2	2
-----	-----	-----	10	17	2.2	1,940	.12	.07	1.9	39
-----	-----	-----	8	13	1.6	1,460	.09	.05	1.5	29
-----	-----	-----	8	54	.6	Trace	.06	.08	.5	34
-----	-----	-----	5	252	1.5	8,270	.15	.33	.7	68
-----	-----	-----	18	8	.4	50	.04	.02	.1	3

TABLE 1.—NUTRITIVE VALUES OF

[Dashes in the columns for nutrients show that no suitable value could be found although

Food, approximate measure, and weight (in grams)			Water	Food energy	Protein	Fat
FRUITS AND FRUIT PRODUCTS—Con.						
		Grams	*Percent*	*Calories*	*Grams*	*Grams*
249	Apple juice, bottled or canned.	1 cup_____ 248	88	120	Trace	Trace
	Applesauce, canned:					
250	Sweetened_____	1 cup_____ 255	76	230	1	Trace
251	Unsweetened or artificially sweetened.	1 cup_____ 244	88	100	1	Trace
	Apricots:					
252	Raw (about 12 per lb.) [5]	3 apricots____ 114	85	55	1	Trace
253	Canned in heavy sirup__	1 cup_____ 259	77	220	2	Trace
254	Dried, uncooked (40 halves per cup).	1 cup_____ 150	25	390	8	1
255	Cooked, unsweetened, fruit and liquid.	1 cup_____ 285	76	240	5	1
256	Apricot nectar, canned___	1 cup_____ 251	85	140	1	Trace
	Avocados, whole fruit, raw: [5]					
257	California (mid- and late-winter; diam. 3⅛ in.).	1 avocado___ 284	74	370	5	37
258	Florida (late summer, fall; diam. 3⅝ in.).	1 avocado___ 454	78	390	4	33
259	Bananas, raw, medium size.[5]	1 banana____ 175	76	100	1	Trace
260	Banana flakes_____	1 cup_____ 100	3	340	4	1
261	Blackberries, raw_____	1 cup_____ 144	84	85	2	1
262	Blueberries, raw_____	1 cup_____ 140	83	85	1	1
263	Cantaloups, raw; medium, 5-inch diameter about 1⅔ pounds.[5]	½ melon____ 385	91	60	1	Trace
264	Cherries, canned, red, sour, pitted, water pack.	1 cup_____ 244	88	105	2	Trace

THE EDIBLE PART OF FOODS—Continued

there is reason to believe that a measurable amount of the nutrient may be present]

Fatty acids			Carbo-hydrate	Cal-cium	Iron	Vita-min A value	Thia-min	Ribo-flavin	Niacin	Ascor-bic acid
Satu-rated (total)	Unsaturated									
	Oleic	Lin-oleic								
Grams	*Grams*	*Grams*	*Grams*	*Milli-grams*	*Milli-grams*	*Inter-national units*	*Milli-grams*	*Milli-grams*	*Milli-grams*	*Milli-grams*
------	------	------	30	15	1.5	-------	.02	.05	.2	2
------	------	------	61	10	1.3	100	.05	.03	.1	[8] 3
------	------	------	26	10	1.2	100	.05	.02	.1	[8] 2
------	------	------	14	18	.5	2,890	.03	.04	.7	10
------	------	------	57	28	.8	4,510	.05	.06	.9	10
------	------	------	100	100	8.2	16,350	.02	.23	4.9	19
------	------	------	62	63	5.1	8,550	.01	.13	2.8	8
------	------	------	37	23	.5	2,380	.03	.03	.5	[8] 8
7	17	5	13	22	1.3	630	.24	.43	3.5	30
7	15	4	27	30	1.8	880	.33	.61	4.9	43
------	------	------	26	10	.8	230	.06	.07	.8	12
------	------	------	89	32	2.8	760	.18	.24	2.8	7
------	------	------	19	46	1.3	290	.05	.06	.5	30
------	------	------	21	21	1.4	140	.04	.08	.6	20
------	------	------	14	27	.8	[9] 6,540	.08	.06	1.2	63
------	------	------	26	37	.7	1,660	.07	.05	.5	12

TABLE 1.—NUTRITIVE VALUES OF

[Dashes in the columns for nutrients show that no suitable value could be found although

	Food, approximate measure, and weight (in grams)		Water	Food energy	Pro- tein	Fat
	FRUITS AND FRUIT PRODUCTS—Con.					
		Grams	Per- cent	Calo- ries	Grams	Grams
265	Cranberry juice cocktail, 1 cup_____ canned.	250	83	165	Trace	Trace
266	Cranberry sauce, sweet- 1 cup_____ ened, canned, strained.	277	62	405	Trace	1
267	Dates, pitted, cut_____ 1 cup_____	178	22	490	4	1
268	Figs, dried, large, 2 by 1 fig_____ 1 in.	21	23	60	1	Trace
269	Fruit cocktail, canned, 1 cup_____ in heavy sirup.	256	80	195	1	Trace
	Grapefruit:					
	Raw, medium, 3¾-in. diam.[5]					
270	White_____ ½ grape- fruit.	241	89	45	1	Trace
271	Pink or red _____ ½ grape- fruit.	241	89	50	1	Trace
272	Canned, sirup pack____ 1 cup_____	254	81	180	2	Trace
	Grapefruit juice:					
273	Fresh_____ 1 cup_____	246	90	95	1	Trace
	Canned, white:					
274	Unsweetened_____ 1 cup_____	247	89	100	1	Trace
275	Sweetened_____ 1 cup_____	250	86	130	1	Trace
	Frozen, concentrate, unsweetened:					
276	Undiluted, can, 6 1 can_____ fluid ounces.	207	62	300	4	1
277	Diluted with 1 cup_____ 3 parts water, by volume.	247	89	100	1	Trace
278	Dehydrated crystals___ 4 oz._____	113	1	410	6	1
279	Prepared with water 1 cup_____ (1 pound yields about 1 gallon).	247	90	100	1	Trace

THE EDIBLE PART OF FOODS—Continued

there is reason to believe that a measurable amount of the nutrient may be present]

Fatty acids			Carbo-hy-drate	Cal-cium	Iron	Vita-min A value	Thia-min	Ribo-flavin	Niacin	Ascor-bic acid
Satu-rated (total)	Unsaturated									
	Oleic	Lin-oleic								
Grams	*Grams*	*Grams*	*Grams*	*Milli-grams*	*Milli-grams*	*Inter-national units*	*Milli-grams*	*Milli-grams*	*Milli-grams*	*Milli-grams*
------	------	------	42	13	.8	Trace	.03	.03	.1	[10] 40
------	------	------	104	17	.6	60	.03	.03	.1	6
------	------	------	130	105	5.3	90	.16	.17	3.9	0
------	------	------	15	26	.6	20	.02	.02	.1	0
------	------	------	50	23	1.0	360	.05	.03	1.3	5
------	------	------	12	19	0.5	10	0.05	0.02	0.2	44
------	------	------	13	20	0.5	540	0.05	0.02	0.2	44
------	------	------	45	33	.8	30	.08	.05	.5	76
------	------	------	23	22	.5	([11])	.09	.04	.4	92
------	------	------	24	20	1.0	20	.07	.04	.4	84
------	------	------	32	20	1.0	20	.07	.04	.4	78
------	------	------	72	70	.8	60	.29	.12	1.4	286
------	------	------	24	25	.2	20	.10	.04	.5	96
------	------	------	102	100	1.2	80	.40	.20	2.0	396
------	------	------	24	22	.2	20	.10	.05	.5	91

TABLE 1.—NUTRITIVE VALUES OF

[Dashes in the columns for nutrients show that no suitable value could be found although

	Food, approximate measure, and weight (in grams)			Water	Food energy	Pro-tein	Fat
				Per-cent	*Calo-ries*	*Grams*	*Grams*

FRUITS AND FRUIT PRODUCTS—Con.

	Food, approximate measure, and weight (in grams)		*Grams*	Water	Food energy	Pro-tein	Fat
	Grapes, raw: [5]						
280	American type (slip skin).	1 cup_____	153	82	65	1	1
281	European type (adherent skin).	1 cup_____	160	81	95	1	Trace
	Grapejuice:						
282	Canned or bottled_____	1 cup_____	253	83	165	1	Trace
	Frozen concentrate, sweetened:						
283	Undiluted, can, 6 fluid ounces.	1 can_____	216	53	395	1	Trace
284	Diluted with 3 parts water, by volume.	1 cup_____	250	86	135	1	Trace
285	Grapejuice drink, canned_	1 cup_____	250	86	135	Trace	Trace
286	Lemons, raw, 2⅛-in. diam., size 165.[5] Used for juice.	1 lemon_____	110	90	20	1	Trace
287	Lemon juice, raw_____	1 cup_____	244	91	60	1	Trace
	Lemonade concentrate:						
288	Frozen, 6 fl. oz. per can_	1 can_____	219	48	430	Trace	Trace
289	Diluted with 4⅓ parts water, by volume.	1 cup_____	248	88	110	Trace	Trace
	Lime juice:						
290	Fresh_____	1 cup_____	246	90	65	1	Trace
291	Canned, unsweetened__	1 cup_____	246	90	65	1	Trace
	Limeade concentrate, frozen:						
292	Undiluted, can, 6 fluid ounces.	1 can_____	218	50	410	Trace	Trace
293	Diluted with 4⅓ parts water, by volume.	1 cup_____	247	90	100	Trace	Trace

THE EDIBLE PART OF FOODS—Continued

there is reason to believe that a measurable amount of the nutrient may be present]

Fatty acids			Carbo-hy-drate	Cal-cium	Iron	Vita-min A value	Thia-min	Ribo-flavin	Niacin	Ascor-bic acid
Satu-rated (total)	Unsaturated									
	Oleic	Lin-oleic								
Grams	*Grams*	*Grams*	*Grams*	*Milli-grams*	*Milli-grams*	*Inter-national units*	*Milli-grams*	*Milli-grams*	*Milli-grams*	*Milli-grams*
------	------	------	15	15	.4	100	.05	.03	.2	3
------	------	------	25	17	.6	140	.07	.04	.4	6
------	------	------	42	28	.8	------	.10	.05	.5	Trace
------	------	------	100	22	.9	40	.13	.22	1.5	(12)
------	------	------	33	8	.3	10	.05	.08	.5	(12)
------	------	------	35	8	.3	------	.03	.03	.3	(12)
------	------	------	6	19	.4	10	.03	.01	.1	39
------	------	------	20	17	.5	50	.07	.02	.2	112
------	------	------	112	9	.4	40	.04	.07	.7	66
------	------	------	28	2	Trace	Trace	Trace	.02	.2	17
------	------	------	22	22	.5	20	.05	.02	.2	79
------	------	------	22	22	.5	20	.05	.02	.2	52
------	------	------	108	11	.2	Trace	.02	.02	.2	26
------	------	------	27	2	Trace	Trace	Trace	Trace	Trace	5

TABLE 1.—NUTRITIVE VALUES OF

[Dashes in the columns for nutrients show that no suitable value could be found although

	Food, approximate measure, and weight (in grams)			Water	Food energy	Pro- tein	Fat
	FRUITS AND FRUIT PRODUCTS—Con.						
			Grams	*Per- cent*	*Calo- ries*	*Grams*	*Grams*
294	Oranges, raw, 2⅝-in. diam., all commercial, varieties.[5]	1 orange_____	180	86	65	1	Trace
295	Orange juice, fresh, all varieties.	1 cup_____	248	88	110	2	1
296	Canned, unsweetened__	1 cup_____	249	87	120	2	Trace
	Frozen concentrate:						
297	Undiluted, can, 6 fluid ounces.	1 can_____	213	55	360	5	Trace
298	Diluted with 3 parts water, by volume.	1 cup_____	249	87	120	2	Trace
299	Dehydrated crystals____	4 oz._____	113	1	430	6	2
300	Prepared with water (1 pound yields about 1 gallon).	1 cup_____	248	88	115	2	1
301	Orange-apricot juice drink	1 cup_____	249	87	125	1	Trace
	Orange and grapefruit juice:						
	Frozen concentrate:						
302	Undiluted, can, 6 fluid ounces.	1 can_____	210	59	330	4	1
303	Diluted with 3 parts water, by volume.	1 cup_____	248	88	110	1	Trace
304	Papayas, raw, ½-inch cubes.	1 cup_____	182	89	70	1	Trace
	Peaches:						
	Raw:						
305	Whole, medium, 2- inch diameter, about 4 per pound.[5]	1 peach_____	114	89	35	1	Trace

THE EDIBLE PART OF FOODS—Continued

there is reason to believe that a measurable amount of the nutrient may be present]

Fatty acids			Carbo-hy-drate	Cal-cium	Iron	Vita-min A value	Thia-min	Ribo-flavin	Niacin	Ascor-bic acid
Satu-rated (total)	Unsaturated									
	Oleic	Lin-oleic								
Grams	*Grams*	*Grams*	*Grams*	*Milli-grams*	*Milli-grams*	*Inter-national units*	*Milli-grams*	*Milli-grams*	*Milli-grams*	*Milli-grams*
------	------	------	16	54	.5	260	.13	.05	.5	66
------	------	------	26	27	.5	500	.22	.07	1.0	124
------	------	------	28	25	1.0	500	.17	.05	.7	100
------	------	------	87	75	.9	1,620	.68	.11	2.8	360
------	------	------	29	25	.2	550	.22	.02	1.0	120
------	------	------	100	95	1.9	1,900	.76	.24	3.3	408
------	------	------	27	25	.5	500	.20	.07	1.0	109
------	------	------	32	12	.2	1,440	.05	.02	.5	[10] 40
------	------	------	78	61	0.8	800	0.48	0.06	2.3	302
------	------	------	26	20	.2	270	.16	.02	.8	102
------	------	------	18	36	.5	3,190	.07	.08	.5	102
------	------	------	10	9	.5	[13]1,320	.02	.05	1.0	7

TABLE 1.—NUTRITIVE VALUES OF

[Dashes in the columns for nutrients show that no suitable value could be found although

	Food, approximate measure, and weight (in grams)		Water	Food energy	Pro-tein	Fat
		Grams	Per-cent	Calo-ries	Grams	Grams
	FRUITS AND FRUIT PRODUCTS—Con.					
306	Sliced_____ 1 cup_____	168	89	65	1	Trace
	Canned, yellow-fleshed, solids and liquid:					
	Sirup pack, heavy:					
307	Halves or slices____ 1 cup_____	257	79	200	1	Trace
308	Water pack_____ 1 cup_____	245	91	75	1	Trace
309	Dried, uncooked_____ 1 cup_____	160	25	420	5	1
310	Cooked, unsweet- 1 cup_____ ened, 10–12 halves and juice.	270	77	220	3	1
	Frozen:					
311	Carton, 12 ounces, 1 carton_____ not thawed.	340	76	300	1	Trace
	Pears:					
312	Raw, 3 by 2½-inch 1 pear_____ diameter.[5]	182	83	100	1	1
	Canned, solids and liquid:					
	Sirup pack, heavy:					
313	Halves or slices____ 1 cup_____	255	80	195	1	1
	Pineapple:					
314	Raw, diced_____ 1 cup_____	140	85	75	1	Trace
	Canned, heavy sirup pack, solids and liquid:					
315	Crushed_____ 1 cup_____	260	80	195	1	Trace
316	Sliced, slices and 2 small or juice. 1 large.	122	80	90	Trace	Trace
317	Pineapple juice, canned___ 1 cup_____	249	86	135	1	Trace
	Plums, all except prunes:					
318	Raw, 2-inch diameter, 1 plum_____ about 2 ounces.[5]	60	87	25	Trace	Trace
	Canned, sirup pack (Italian prunes):					
319	Plums (with pits) 1 cup_____ and juice.[5]	256	77	205	1	Trace

THE EDIBLE PART OF FOODS—Continued

there is reason to believe that a measurable amount of the nutrient may be present]

Fatty acids			Carbo-hy-drate	Cal-cium	Iron	Vita-min A value	Thia-min	Ribo-flavin	Niacin	Ascor-bic acid
Satu-rated (total)	Unsaturated									
	Oleic	Lin-oleic								
Grams	*Grams*	*Grams*	*Grams*	*Milli-grams*	*Milli-grams*	*Inter-national units*	*Milli-grams*	*Milli-grams*	*Milli-grams*	*Milli-grams*
------	------	------	16	15	.8	[13]2,230	.03	.08	1.6	12
------	------	------	52	10	.8	1,100	.02	.06	1.4	7
------	------	------	20	10	.7	1,100	.02	.06	1.4	7
------	------	------	109	77	9.6	6,240	.02	.31	8.5	28
------	------	------	58	41	5.1	3,290	.01	.15	4.2	6
------	------	------	77	14	1.7	2,210	.03	.14	2.4	[14] 135
------	------	------	25	13	.5	30	.04	.07	.2	7
------	------	------	50	13	.5	Trace	.03	.05	.3	4
------	------	------	19	24	.7	100	.12	.04	.3	24
------	------	------	50	29	.8	120	.20	.06	.5	17
------	------	------	24	13	.4	50	.09	.03	.2	8
------	------	------	34	37	.7	120	.12	.04	.5	[8] 22
------	------	------	7	7	.3	140	.02	.02	.3	3
------	------	------	53	22	2.2	2,970	.05	.05	.9	4

TABLE 1.—NUTRITIVE VALUES OF

[Dashes in the columns for nutrients show that no suitable value could be found although

	Food, approximate measure, and weight (in grams)		Water	Food energy	Pro- tein	Fat
	FRUITS AND FRUIT PRODUCTS—Con.	*Grams*	*Per- cent*	*Calo- ries*	*Grams*	*Grams*
	Prunes, dried, "softenized", medium:					
320	Uncooked [5] _ _ _ _ _ _ _ _ _ _ _ _ 4 prunes _ _ _ _ _	32	28	70	1	Trace
321	Cooked, unsweetened, 1 cup _ _ _ _ _ _ _ _ 17–18 prunes and ⅓ cup liquid.[5]	270	66	295	2	1
322	Prune juice, canned or · 1 cup _ _ _ _ _ _ _ _ bottled.	256	80	200	1	Trace
	Raisins, seedless:					
323	Packaged, ½ oz. or 1 pkg. _ _ _ _ _ _ _ _ 1½ tbsp. per pkg.	14	18	40	Trace	Trace
324	Cup, pressed down _ _ _ _ 1 cup _ _ _ _ _ _ _	165	18	480	4	Trace
	Raspberries, red:					
325	Raw _ _ _ _ _ _ _ _ _ _ _ _ _ _ _ _ _ 1 cup _ _ _ _ _ _ _	123	84	70	1	1
326	Frozen, 10-ounce car- 1 carton _ _ _ _ _ ton, not thawed.	284	74	275	2	1
327	Rhubarb, cooked, sugar 1 cup _ _ _ _ _ _ _ _ added.	272	63	385	1	Trace
	Strawberries:					
328	Raw, capped _ _ _ _ _ _ _ _ _ _ 1 cup _ _ _ _ _ _ _	149	90	55	1	1
329	Frozen, 10-ounce car- 1 carton _ _ _ _ _ ton, not thawed.	284	71	310	1	1
330	Tangerines, raw, medium, 1 tangerine _ _ 2⅜-in. diam., size 176.[5]	116	87	40	1	Trace
331	Tangerine juice, canned, 1 cup _ _ _ _ _ _ _ _ sweetened.	249	87	125	1	1
332	Watermelon, raw, wedge, 1 wedge _ _ _ _ _ _ 4 by 8 inches (¹⁄₁₆ of 10 by 16-inch melon, about 2 pounds with rind).[5]	925	93	115	2	1

THE EDIBLE PART OF FOODS—Continued

there is reason to believe that a measurable amount of the nutrient may be present]

Fatty acids			Carbo-hy-drate	Cal-cium	Iron	Vita-min A value	Thia-min	Ribo-flavin	Niacin	Ascor-bic acid
Satu-rated (total)	Unsaturated									
	Oleic	Lin-oleic								
Grams	*Grams*	*Grams*	*Grams*	*Milli-grams*	*Milli-grams*	*Inter-national units*	*Milli-grams*	*Milli-grams*	*Milli-grams*	*Milli-grams*
_____	_____	_____	18	14	1.1	440	.02	.04	.4	1
_____	_____	_____	78	60	4.5	1,860	.08	.18	1.7	2
_____	_____	_____	49	36	10.5	_____	.03	.03	1.0	[8] 5
_____	_____	_____	11	9	.5	Trace	.02	.01	.1	Trace
_____	_____	_____	128	102	5.8	30	.18	.13	.8	2
_____	_____	_____	17	27	1.1	160	.04	.11	1.1	31
_____	_____	_____	70	37	1.7	200	.06	.17	1.7	59
_____	_____	_____	98	212	1.6	220	.06	.15	.7	17
_____	_____	_____	13	31	1.5	90	.04	.10	1.0	88
_____	_____	_____	79	40	2.0	90	.06	.17	1.5	150
_____	_____	_____	10	34	.3	360	.05	.02	.1	27
_____	_____	_____	30	45	.5	1,050	.15	.05	.2	55
_____	_____	_____	27	30	2.1	2,510	.13	.13	.7	30

TABLE 1.—NUTRITIVE VALUES OF

[Dashes in the columns for nutrients show that no suitable value could be found although

	Food, approximate measure, and weight (in grams)			Water	Food energy	Pro-tein	Fat
			Grams	*Per-cent*	*Calo-ries*	*Grams*	*Grams*
	GRAIN PRODUCTS						
	Bagel, 3-in. diam.:						
333	Egg_____	1 bagel_____	55	32	165	6	2
334	Water_____	1 bagel_____	55	29	165	6	2
335	Barley, pearled, light, uncooked.	1 cup_____	200	11	700	16	2
336	Biscuits, baking powder from home recipe with enriched flour, 2-in. diam.	1 biscuit_____	28	27	105	2	5
337	Biscuits, baking powder from mix, 2-in. diam.	1 biscuit_____	28	28	90	2	3
338	Bran flakes (40% bran), added thiamin and iron.	1 cup_____	35	3	105	4	1
339	Bran flakes with raisins, added thiamin and iron.	1 cup_____	50	7	145	4	1
	Breads:						
340	Boston brown bread, slice 3 by ¾ in.	1 slice_____	48	45	100	3	1
	Cracked-wheat bread:						
341	Loaf, 1 lb._____	1 loaf_____	454	35	1,190	40	10
342	Slice, 18 slices per loaf.	1 slice_____	25	35	65	2	1
	French or vienna bread:						
343	Enriched, 1 lb. loaf__	1 loaf_____	454	31	1,315	41	14
344	Unenriched, 1 lb. loaf.	1 loaf_____	454	31	1,315	41	14
	Italian bread:						
345	Enriched, 1 lb. loaf__	1 loaf_____	454	32	1,250	41	4
346	Unenriched, 1 lb. loaf.	1 loaf_____	454	32	1,250	41	4

THE EDIBLE PART OF FOODS—Continued

there is reason to believe that a measurable amount of the nutrient may be present]

Fatty acids			Carbo-hy-drate	Cal-cium	Iron	Vita-min A value	Thia-min	Ribo-flavin	Niacin	Ascor-bic acid
Satu-rated (total)	Unsaturated									
	Oleic	Lin-oleic								
Grams	*Grams*	*Grams*	*Grams*	*Milli-grams*	*Milli-grams*	*Inter-national units*	*Milli-grams*	*Milli-grams*	*Milli-grams*	*Milli-grams*
------	------	------	28	9	1.2	30	0.14	0.10	1.2	0
------	------	------	30	8	1.2	0	.15	.11	1.4	0
Trace	1	1	158	32	4.0	0	.24	.10	6.2	0
1	2	1	13	34	.4	Trace	.06	.06	.1	Trace
1	1	1	15	19	.6	Trace	.08	.07	.6	Trace
------	------	------	28	25	12.3	0	.14	.06	2.2	0
------	------	------	40	28	13.5	Trace	.16	.07	2.7	0
------	------	------	22	43	.9	0	.05	.03	.6	0
2	5	2	236	399	5.0	Trace	.53	.41	5.9	Trace
------	------	------	13	22	.3	Trace	.03	.02	.3	Trace
3	8	2	251	195	10.0	Trace	1.27	1.00	11.3	Trace
3	8	2	251	195	3.2	Trace	.36	.36	3.6	Trace
Trace	1	2	256	77	10.0	0	1.32	.91	11.8	0
Trace	1	2	256	77	3.2	0	.41	.27	3.6	0

TABLE 1.—NUTRITIVE VALUES OF

[Dashes in the columns for nutrients show that no suitable value could be found although

	Food, approximate measure, and weight (in grams)			Water	Food energy	Pro-tein	Fat
			Grams	Per-cent	Calo-ries	Grams	Grams
	GRAIN PRODUCTS—Continued						
	Raisin bread:						
347	Loaf, 1 lb._____	1 loaf_____	454	35	1,190	30	13
348	Slice, 18 slices per loaf.	1 slice_____	25	35	65	2	1
	Rye bread:						
	American, light (⅓ rye, ⅔ wheat):						
349	Loaf, 1 lb._____	1 loaf_____	454	36	1,100	41	5
350	Slice, 18 slices per loaf.	1 slice_____	25	36	60	2	Trace
351	Pumpernickel, loaf, 1 lb.	1 loaf_____	454	34	1,115	41	5
	White bread, enriched: [15]						
	Soft-crumb type:						
352	Loaf, 1 lb._____	1 loaf_____	454	36	1,225	39	15
353	Slice, 18 slices per loaf.	1 slice_____	25	36	70	2	1
354	Slice, toasted____	1 slice_____	22	25	70	2	1
355	Slice, 22 slices per loaf.	1 slice_____	20	36	55	2	1
356	Slice, toasted____	1 slice_____	17	25	55	2	1
357	Loaf, 1½ lbs._____	1 loaf_____	680	36	1,835	59	22
358	Slice, 24 slices per loaf.	1 slice_____	28	36	75	2	1
359	Slice, toasted____	1 slice_____	24	25	75	2	1
360	Slice, 28 slices per loaf.	1 slice_____	24	36	65	2	1
361	Slice, toasted____	1 slice_____	21	25	65	2	1
	Firm-crumb type:						
362	Loaf, 1 lb._____	1 loaf_____	454	35	1,245	41	17
363	Slice, 20 slices per loaf.	1 slice_____	23	35	65	2	1

THE EDIBLE PART OF FOODS—Continued

there is reason to believe that a measurable amount of the nutrient may be present]

Fatty acids			Carbo-hy-drate	Cal-cium	Iron	Vita-min A value	Thia-min	Ribo-flavin	Niacin	Ascor-bic acid
Satu-rated (total)	Unsaturated									
	Oleic	Lin-oleic								
Grams	*Grams*	*Grams*	*Grams*	*Milli-grams*	*Milli-grams*	*Inter-national units*	*Milli-grams*	*Milli-grams*	*Milli-grams*	*Milli-grams*
3	8	2	243	322	5.9	Trace	.23	.41	3.2	Trace
--	--	--	13	18	.3	Trace	.01	.02	.2	Trace
--	--	--	236	340	7.3	0	.82	.32	6.4	0
--	--	--	13	19	.4	0	.05	.02	.4	0
--	--	--	241	381	10.9	0	1.04	.64	5.4	0
3	8	2	229	381	11.3	Trace	1.13	.95	10.9	Trace
--	--	--	13	21	.6	Trace	.06	.05	.6	Trace
--	--	--	13	21	.6	Trace	.06	.05	.6	Trace
--	--	--	10	17	.5	Trace	.05	.04	.5	Trace
--	--	--	10	17	.5	Trace	.05	.04	.5	Trace
5	12	3	343	571	17.0	Trace	1.70	1.43	16.3	Trace
--	--	--	14	24	.7	Trace	.07	.06	.7	Trace
--	--	--	14	24	.7	Trace	.07	.06	.7	Trace
--	--	--	12	20	.6	Trace	.06	.05	.6	Trace
--	--	--	12	20	.6	Trace	.06	.05	.6	Trace
4	10	2	228	435	11.3	Trace	1.22	.91	10.9	Trace
--	--	--	12	22	.6	Trace	.06	.05	.6	Trace

TABLE 1.—NUTRITIVE VALUES OF

[Dashes show that no basis could be found for imputing a value although there was

	Food, approximate measure, and weight (in grams)	Water	Food energy	Pro-tein	Fat
	GRAIN PRODUCTS—Continued				
		Grams	Per-cent	Calo-ries	Grams	Grams
364	Slice, toasted____ 1 slice_____ 20	24	65	2	1
365	Loaf, 2 lbs._____ 1 loaf_____ 907	35	2,495	82	34
366	Slice, 34 slices 1 slice_____ 27 per loaf.	35	75	2	1
367	Slice, toasted____ 1 slice_____ 23	35	75	2	1
	Whole-wheat bread, soft-crumb type:				
368	Loaf, 1 lb._____ 1 loaf_____ 454	36	1,095	41	12
369	Slice, 16 slices per 1 slice_____ 28 loaf.	36	65	3	1
370	Slice, toasted_____ 1 slice_____ 24	24	65	3	1
	Whole-wheat bread, firm-crumb type:				
371	Loaf, 1 lb._____ 1 loaf_____ 454	36	1,100	48	14
372	Slice, 18 slices per 1 slice_____ 25 loaf.	36	60	3	1
373	Slice, toasted_____ 1 slice_____ 21	24	60	3	1
374	Breadcrumbs, dry, grated_ 1 cup_____ 100	6	390	13	5
375	Buckwheat flour, light, 1 cup_____ 98 sifted.	12	340	6	1
376	Bulgur, canned, seasoned_ 1 cup_____ 135	56	245	8	4
	Cakes made from cake mixes:				
	Angelfood:				
377	Whole cake_____ 1 cake_____ 635	34	1,645	36	1
378	Piece, 1/12 of 10-in. 1 piece_____ 53 diam. cake.	34	135	3	Trace
	Cupcakes, small, 2½ in. diam.:				
379	Without icing_____ 1 cupcake___ 25	26	90	1	3
380	With chocolate icing_ 1 cupcake___ 36	22	130	2	5
	Devil's food, 2-layer, with chocolate icing:				
381	Whole cake_____ 1 cake_____1,107	24	3,755	49	136
382	Piece, 1/16 of 9-in. 1 piece_____ 69 diam. cake.	24	235	3	9

THE EDIBLE PART OF FOODS—Continued

some reason to believe that a measurable amount of the constituent might be present]

Fatty acids			Carbo-hy-drate	Cal-cium	Iron	Vita-min A value	Thia-min	Ribo-flavin	Niacin	Ascor-bic acid
Satu-rated (total)	Unsaturated									
	Oleic	Lin-oleic								
Grams	*Grams*	*Grams*	*Grams*	*Milli-grams*	*Milli-grams*	*Inter-national units*	*Milli-grams*	*Milli-grams*	*Milli-grams*	*Milli-grams*
			12	22	.6	Trace	.06	.05	.6	Trace
8	20	4	455	871	22.7	Trace	2.45	1.81	21.8	Trace
			14	26	.7	Trace	.07	.05	.6	Trace
			14	26	.7	Trace	.07	.05	.6	Trace
2	6	2	224	381	13.6	Trace	1.36	.45	12.7	Trace
			14	24	.8	Trace	.09	.03	.8	Trace
			14	24	.8	Trace	.09	.03	.8	Trace
3	6	3	216	449	13.6	Trace	1.18	0.54	12.7	Trace
			12	25	.8	Trace	.06	.03	.7	Trace
			12	25	.8	Trace	.06	.03	.7	Trace
1	2	1	73	122	3.6	Trace	.22	.30	3.5	Trace
			78	11	1.0	0	.08	.04	.4	0
			44	27	1.9	0	.08	.05	4.1	0
			377	603	1.9	0	.03	.70	.6	0
			32	50	.2	0	Trace	.06	.1	0
1	1	1	14	40	.1	40	.01	.03	.1	Trace
2	2	1	21	47	.3	60	.01	.04	.1	Trace
54	58	16	645	653	8.9	1,660	.33	.89	3.3	1
3	4	1	40	41	.6	100	.02	.06	.2	Trace

TABLE 1.—NUTRITIVE VALUES OF

[Dashes show that no basis could be found for imputing a value although there was

Food, approximate measure, and weight (in grams)			Water	Food energy	Pro-tein	Fat
			Per-cent	*Calo-ries*	*Grams*	*Grams*
GRAIN PRODUCTS—Continued		*Grams*				
383	Cupcake, small, 2½ in. diam.	1 cupcake___ 35	24	120	2	4
	Gingerbread:					
384	Whole cake_____ 1 cake_____	570	37	1,575	18	39
385	Piece, ⅑ of 8-in. square cake.	1 piece_____ 63	37	175	2	4
	White, 2-layer, with chocolate icing:					
386	Whole cake_____ 1 cake_____	1,140	21	4,000	45	122
387	Piece, ¹⁄₁₆ of 9-in. diam. cake.	1 piece_____ 71	21	250	3	8
	Cakes made from home recipes: [16]					
388	Boston cream pie; piece ¹⁄₁₂ of 8-in. diam.	1 piece_____ 69	35	210	4	6
	Fruitcake, dark, made with enriched flour:					
389	Loaf, 1-lb._____ 1 loaf_____	454	18	1,720	22	69
390	Slice, 1/30 of 8-in. loaf.	1 slice_____ 15	18	55	1	2
	Plain sheet cake:					
	Without icing:					
391	Whole cake_____ 1 cake_____	777	25	2,830	35	108
392	Piece, ⅑ of 9-in. square cake.	1 piece_____ 86	25	315	4	12
393	With boiled white icing, piece, ⅑ of 9-in. square cake.	1 piece_____ 114	23	400	4	12
	Pound:					
394	Loaf, 8½ by 3½ by 3in.	1 loaf_____ 514	17	2,430	29	152
395	Slice, ½-in. thick____ 1 slice_____	30	17	140	2	9

THE EDIBLE PART OF FOODS—Continued

some reason to believe that a measurable amount of the constituent might be present]

Fatty acids			Carbohydrate	Calcium	Iron	Vitamin A value	Thiamin	Riboflavin	Niacin	Ascorbic acid
Saturated (total)	Unsaturated									
	Oleic	Linoleic								
Grams	*Grams*	*Grams*	*Grams*	*Milligrams*	*Milligrams*	*International units*	*Milligrams*	*Milligrams*	*Milligrams*	*Milligrams*
1	2	Trace	20	21	.3	50	.01	.03	.1	Trace
10	19	9	291	513	9.1	Trace	.17	.51	4.6	2
1	2	1	32	57	1.0	Trace	.02	.06	.5	Trace
45	54	17	716	1,129	5.7	680	.23	.91	2.3	2
3	3	1	45	70	.4	40	.01	.06	.1	Trace
2	3	1	34	46	.3	140	.02	.08	.1	Trace
15	37	13	271	327	11.8	540	.59	.64	3.6	2
Trace	1	Trace	9	11	.4	20	.02	.02	.1	Trace
30	52	21	434	497	3.1	1,320	.16	.70	1.6	2
3	6	2	48	55	.3	150	.02	.08	.2	Trace
3	6	2	71	56	.3	150	.02	.08	.2	Trace
34	68	17	242	108	4.1	1,440	.15	.46	1.0	0
2	4	1	14	6	.2	80	.01	.03	.1	0

TABLE 1.—NUTRITIVE VALUES OF

[Dashes in the columns for nutrients show that no suitable value could be found although

	Food, approximate measure, and weight (in grams)	Water	Food energy	Pro-tein	Fat
	GRAIN PRODUCTS—Continued				
	Sponge:	Grams	Per-cent	Calo-ries	Grams	Grams
396	Whole cake_____ 1 cake_____ 790	32	2,345	60	45
397	Piece, ¹⁄₁₂ of 10-in. 1 piece_____ 66	32	195	5	4
	diam. cake.				
	Yellow, 2-layer, without icing:				
398	Whole cake_____ 1 cake_____ 870	24	3,160	39	111
399	Piece, ¹⁄₁₆ of 9-in. 1 piece_____ 54	24	200	2	7
	diam. cake.				
	Yellow, 2-layer, with chocolate icing:				
400	Whole cake_____ 1 cake_____1,203	21	4,390	51	156
401	Piece, ¹⁄₁₆ of 9-in. 1 piece_____ 75	21	275	3	10
	diam. cake.				
	Cake icings. See Sugars, Sweets.				
	Cookies:				
	Brownies with nuts:				
402	Made from home 1 brownie____ 20 recipe with en-riched flour.	10	95	1	6
403	Made from mix_____ 1 brownie____ 20	11	85	1	4
	Chocolate chip:				
404	Made from home 1 cookie_____ 10 recipe with en-riched flour.	3	50	1	3
405	Commercial_____ 1 cookie_____ 10	3	50	1	2
406	Fig bars, commercial___ 1 cookie_____ 14	14	50	1	1
407	Sandwich, chocolate or 1 cookie_____ 10 vanilla, commercial.	2	50	1	2
	Corn flakes, added nutrients:				
408	Plain_____ 1 cup_____ 25	4	100	2	Trace
409	Sugar-covered_____ 1 cup_____ 40	2	155	2	Trace

THE EDIBLE PART OF FOODS—Continued

there is reason to believe that a measurable amount of the nutrient may be present]

Fatty acids			Carbo-hy-drate	Cal-cium	Iron	Vita-min A value	Thia-min	Ribo-flavin	Niacin	Ascor-bic acid
Satu-rated (total)	Unsaturated									
	Oleic	Lin-oleic								
Grams	*Grams*	*Grams*	*Grams*	*Milli-grams*	*Milli-grams*	*Inter-national units*	*Milli-grams*	*Milli-grams*	*Milli-grams*	*Milli-grams*
14	20	4	427	237	9.5	3,560	.40	1.11	1.6	Trace
1	2	Trace	36	20	.8	300	.03	.09	.1	Trace
31	53	22	506	618	3.5	1,310	.17	.70	1.7	2
2	3	1	32	39	.2	80	.01	.04	.1	Trace
55	69	23	727	818	7.2	1,920	.24	.96	2.4	Trace
3	4	1	45	51	.5	120	.02	.06	.2	Trace
1	3	1	10	8	.4	40	.04	.02	.1	Trace
1	2	1	13	9	.4	20	.03	.02	.1	Trace
1	1	1	6	4	0.2	10	0.01	0.01	0.1	Trace
1	1	Trace	7	4	.2	10	Trace	Trace	Trace	Trace
			11	11	.2	20	Trace	.01	.1	Trace
1	1	Trace	7	2	.1	0	Trace	Trace	.1	0
			21	4	.4	0	.11	.02	.5	0
			36	5	.4	0	.16	.02	.8	0

TABLE 1.—NUTRITIVE VALUES OF

[Dashes in the columns for nutrients show that no suitable value could be found although

	Food, approximate measure, and weight (in grams)			Water	Food energy	Pro-tein	Fat
	GRAIN PRODUCTS—Continued						
			Grams	*Per-cent*	*Calo-ries*	*Grams*	*Grams*
	Corn (hominy) grits, degermed, cooked:						
410	Enriched	1 cup	245	87	125	3	Trace
411	Unenriched	1 cup	245	87	125	3	Trace
	Cornmeal:						
412	Whole-ground, unbolted, dry.	1 cup	122	12	435	11	5
413	Bolted (nearly whole-grain) dry.	1 cup	122	12	440	11	4
	Degermed, enriched:						
414	Dry form	1 cup	138	12	500	11	2
415	Cooked	1 cup	240	88	120	3	1
	Degermed, unenriched:						
416	Dry form	1 cup	138	12	500	11	2
417	Cooked	1 cup	240	88	120	3	1
418	Corn muffins, made with enriched de-germed cornmeal and enriched flour; muffin 2⅜-in. diam.	1 muffin	40	33	125	3	4
419	Corn muffins, made with mix, egg, and milk; muffin 2⅜-in. diam.	1 muffin	40	30	130	3	4
420	Corn, puffed, presweet-ened, added nutrients.	1 cup	30	2	115	1	Trace
421	Corn, shredded, added nutrients.	1 cup	25	3	100	2	Trace
	Crackers:						
422	Graham, 2½-in. square	4 crackers	28	6	110	2	3
423	Saltines	4 crackers	11	4	50	1	1

THE EDIBLE PART OF FOODS—Continued

there is reason to believe that a measurable amount of the nutrient may be present]

Fatty acids			Carbo-hy-drate	Cal-cium	Iron	Vita-min A value	Thia-min	Ribo-flavin	Niacin	Ascor-bic acid
Satu-rated (total)	Unsaturated									
	Oleic	Lin-oleic								
Grams	*Grams*	*Grams*	*Grams*	*Milli-grams*	*Milli-grams*	*Inter-national units*	*Milli-grams*	*Milli-grams*	*Milli-grams*	*Milli-grams*
------	------	------	27	2	.7	[17] 150	.10	.07	1.0	0
------	------	------	27	2	.2	[17] 150	.05	.02	.5	0
1	2	2	90	24	2.9	[17] 620	.46	.13	2.4	0
Trace	1	2	91	21	2.2	[17] 590	.37	.10	2.3	0
------	------	------	108	8	4.0	[17] 610	.61	.36	4.8	0
------	------	------	26	2	1.0	[17] 140	.14	.10	1.2	0
------	------	------	108	8	1.5	[17] 610	.19	.07	1.4	0
------	------	------	26	2	.5	[17] 140	.05	.02	.2	0
2	2	Trace	19	42	.7	[17] 120	.08	.09	.6	Trace
1	2	1	20	96	.6	100	.07	.08	.6	Trace
------	------	------	27	3	.5	0	.13	.05	.6	0
------	------	------	22	1	.6	0	.11	.05	.5	0
------	------	------	21	11	.4	0	.01	.06	.4	0
------	1	------	8	2	.1	0	Trace	Trace	.1	0

TABLE 1.—NUTRITIVE VALUES OF

[Dashes in the columns for nutrients show that no suitable value could be found although

	Food, approximate measure, and weight (in grams)			Water	Food energy	Pro-tein	Fat
			Grams	Per-cent	Calo-ries	Grams	Grams
	GRAIN PRODUCTS						
	Danish pastry, plain (without fruit or nuts):						
424	Packaged ring, 12 ounces.	1 ring_____	340	22	1,435	25	80
425	Round piece, approx. 4¼-in. diam. by 1 in.	1 pastry_____	65	22	275	5	15
426	Ounce_____	1 oz._____	28	22	120	2	7
427	Doughnuts, cake type____	1 doughnut__	32	24	125	1	6
428	Farina, quick-cooking, enriched, cooked.	1 cup_____	245	89	105	3	Trace
	Macaroni, cooked:						
	Enriched:						
429	Cooked, firm stage (undergoes additional cooking in a food mixture).	1 cup_____	130	64	190	6	1
430	Cooked until tender__	1 cup_____	140	72	155	5	1
	Unenriched:						
431	Cooked, firm stage (undergoes additional cooking in a food mixture).	1 cup_____	130	64	190	6	1
432	Cooked until tender__	1 cup_____	140	72	155	5	1
433	Macaroni (enriched) and cheese, baked.	1 cup_____	200	58	430	17	22
434	Canned_____	1 cup_____	240	80	230	9	10
435	Muffins, with enriched white flour; muffin, 3-inch diam.	1 muffin ____	40	38	120	3	4
	Noodles (egg noodles), cooked:						
436	Enriched_____	1 cup_____	160	70	200	7	2
437	Unenriched_____	1 cup_____	160	70	200	7	2

THE EDIBLE PART OF FOODS—Continued

there is reason to believe that a measurable amount of the nutrient may be present]

Fatty acids			Carbo-hydrate	Cal-cium	Iron	Vita-min A value	Thia-min	Ribo-flavin	Niacin	Ascorbic acid
Saturated (total)	Unsaturated									
	Oleic	Linoleic								
Grams	Grams	Grams	Grams	Milligrams	Milligrams	International units	Milligrams	Milligrams	Milligrams	Milligrams
24	37	15	155	170	3.1	1,050	.24	.51	2.7	Trace
5	7	3	30	33	.6	200	.05	.10	.5	Trace
2	3	1	13	14	.3	90	.02	.04	.2	Trace
1	4	Trace	16	13	[18].4	30	[18].05	[18].05	[18].4	Trace
-----	-----	-----	22	147	[19].7	0	[19].12	[19].07	[19]1.0	0
-----	-----	-----	39	14	[19]1.4	0	[19].23	[19].14	[19]1.8	0
-----	-----	-----	32	8	[19]1.3	0	[19].20	[19].11	[19]1.5	0
-----	-----	-----	39	14	.7	0	.03	.03	.5	0
-----	-----	-----	32	11	.6	0	.01	.01	.4	0
10	9	2	40	362	1.8	860	.20	.40	1.8	Trace
4	3	1	26	199	1.0	260	.12	.24	1.0	Trace
1	2	1	17	42	.6	40	.07	.09	.6	Trace
1	1	Trace	37	16	[19]1.4	110	[19].22	[19].13	[19]1.9	0
1	1	Trace	37	16	1.0	110	.05	.03	.6	0

TABLE 1.—NUTRITIVE VALUES OF

[Dashes in the columns for nutrients show that no suitable value could be found although

	Food, approximate measure, and weight (in grams)			Water	Food energy	Pro-tein	Fat
	GRAIN PRODUCTS—Continued						
			Grams	Per-cent	Calo-ries	Grams	Grams
438	Oats (with or without corn) puffed, added nutrients.	1 cup	25	3	100	3	1
439	Oatmeal or rolled oats, cooked.	1 cup	240	87	130	5	2
	Pancakes, 4-inch diam.:						
440	Wheat, enriched flour (home recipe).	1 cake	27	50	60	2	2
441	Buckwheat (made from mix with egg and milk).	1 cake	27	58	55	2	2
442	Plain or buttermilk (made from mix with egg and milk).	1 cake	27	51	60	2	2
	Pie (piecrust made with unenriched flour):						
	Sector, 4-in., 1/7 of 9-in. diam. pie:						
443	Apple (2-crust)	1 sector	135	48	350	3	15
444	Butterscotch (1-crust)	1 sector	130	45	350	6	14
445	Cherry (2-crust)	1 sector	135	47	350	4	15
446	Custard (1-crust)	1 sector	130	58	285	8	14
447	Lemon meringue (1-crust).	1 sector	120	47	305	4	12
448	Mince (2-crust)	1 sector	135	43	365	3	16
449	Pecan (1-crust)	1 sector	118	20	490	6	27
450	Pineapple chiffon (1-crust).	1 sector	93	41	265	6	11
451	Pumpkin (1-crust)	1 sector	130	59	275	5	15
	Piecrust, baked shell for pie made with:						
452	Enriched flour	1 shell	180	15	900	11	60
453	Unenriched flour	1 shell	180	15	900	11	60

THE EDIBLE PART OF FOODS—Continued

there is reason to believe that a measurable amount of the nutrient may be present]

Fatty acids			Carbo-hy-drate	Cal-cium	Iron	Vita-min A value	Thia-min	Ribo-flavin	Niacin	Ascor-bic acid
Satu-rated (total)	Unsaturated									
	Oleic	Lin-oleic								
Grams	*Grams*	*Grams*	*Grams*	*Milli-grams*	*Milli-grams*	*Inter-national units*	*Milli-grams*	*Milli-grams*	*Milli-grams*	*Milli-grams*
------	------	------	19	44	1.2	0	0.24	0.04	0.5	0
------	------	1	23	22	1.4	0	.19	.05	.2	0
Trace	1	Trace	9	27	.4	30	.05	.06	.4	Trace
1	1	Trace	6	59	.4	60	.03	.04	.2	Trace
1	1	Trace	9	58	.3	70	.04	.06	.2	Trace
4	7	3	51	11	.4	40	.03	.03	.5	1
5	6	2	50	98	1.2	340	.04	.13	.3	Trace
4	7	3	52	19	.4	590	.03	.03	.7	Trace
5	6	2	30	125	.8	300	.07	.21	.4	0
4	6	2	45	17	.6	200	.04	.10	.2	4
4	8	3	56	38	1.4	Trace	.09	.05	.5	1
4	16	5	60	55	3.3	190	.19	.08	.4	Trace
3	5	2	36	22	.8	320	.04	.08	.4	1
5	6	2	32	66	.7	3,210	.04	.13	.7	Trace
16	28	12	79	25	3.1	0	.36	.25	3.2	0
16	28	12	79	25	.9	0	.05	.05	.9	0

TABLE 1.—NUTRITIVE VALUES OF

[Dashes in the columns for nutrients show that no suitable value could be found although

	Food, approximate measure, and weight (in grams)			Water	Food energy	Pro-tein	Fat
				Per-cent	Calo-ries	Grams	Grams
	GRAIN PRODUCTS—Continued		Grams				
	Piecrust mix including stick form:						
454	Package, 10-oz., for double crust.	1 pkg_____	284	9	1,480	20	93
455	Pizza (cheese) 5½-in. sector; ⅛ of 14-in. diam. pie.	1 sector_____	75	45	185	7	6
	Popcorn, popped:						
456	Plain, large kernel_____	1 cup_____	6	4	25	1	Trace
457	With oil and salt_____	1 cup_____	9	3	40	1	2
458	Sugar coated_____	1 cup_____	35	4	135	2	1
	Pretzels:						
459	Dutch, twisted_____	1 pretzel____	16	5	60	2	1
460	Thin, twisted_____	1 pretzel____	6	5	25	1	Trace
461	Stick, small, 2¼ inches_	10 sticks____	3	5	10	Trace	Trace
462	Stick, regular, 3⅛ inches.	5 sticks_____	3	5	10	Trace	Trace
	Rice, white:						
	Enriched:						
463	Raw_____	1 cup_____	185	12	670	12	1
464	Cooked_____	1 cup_____	205	73	225	4	Trace
465	Instant, ready-to-serve.	1 cup_____	165	73	180	4	Trace
466	Unenriched, cooked____	1 cup_____	205	73	225	4	Trace
467	Parboiled, cooked_____	1 cup_____	175	73	185	4	Trace
468	Rice, puffed, added nutrients.	1 cup_____	15	4	60	1	Trace
	Rolls, enriched:						
	Cloverleaf or pan:						
469	Home recipe_____	1 roll_____	35	26	120	3	3
470	Commercial_____	1 roll_____	28	31	85	2	2
471	Frankfurter or hamburger.	1 roll_____	40	31	120	3	2

THE EDIBLE PART OF FOODS—Continued

there is reason to believe that a measurable amount of the nutrient may be present]

Fatty acids			Carbo-hydrate	Cal-cium	Iron	Vita-min A value	Thia-min	Ribo-flavin	Niacin	Ascor-bic acid
Satu-rated (total)	Unsaturated									
	Oleic	Lin-oleic								
Grams	*Grams*	*Grams*	*Grams*	*Milli-grams*	*Milli-grams*	*Inter-national units*	*Milli-grams*	*Milli-grams*	*Milli-grams*	*Milli-grams*
23	46	21	141	131	1.4	0	.11	.11	2.0	0
2	3	Trace	27	107	.7	290	.04	.12	.7	4
------	------	------	5	1	.2	------	------	.01	.1	0
1	Trace	Trace	5	1	.2	------	------	.01	.2	0
------	------	------	30	2	.5	------	------	.02	.4	0
------	------	------	12	4	.2	0	Trace	Trace	.1	0
------	------	------	5	1	.1	0	Trace	Trace	Trace	0
------	------	------	2	1	Trace	0	Trace	Trace	Trace	0
------	------	------	2	1	Trace	0	Trace	Trace	Trace	0
------	------	------	149	44	[20]5.4	0	[20].81	[20].06	[20]6.5	0
------	------	------	50	21	[20]1.8	0	[20].23	[20].02	[20]2.1	0
------	------	------	40	5	[20]1.3	0	[20].21	[20]---	[20]1.7	0
------	------	------	50	21	.4	0	.04	.02	.8	0
------	------	------	41	33	[20]1.4	0	[20].19	[20]---	[20]2.1	0
------	------	------	13	3	.3	0	.07	.01	.7	0
1	1	1	20	16	.7	30	.09	.09	.8	Trace
Trace	1	Trace	15	21	.5	Trace	.08	.05	.6	Trace
1	1	1	21	30	.8	Trace	.11	.07	.9	Trace

TABLE 1.—NUTRITIVE VALUES OF

[Dashes in the columns for nutrients show that no suitable value could be found although

	Food, approximate measure, and weight (in grams)			Water	Food energy	Pro-tein	Fat
	GRAIN PRODUCTS						
			Grams	*Per-cent*	*Calo-ries*	*Grams*	*Grams*
472	Hard, round or rectangular.	1 roll_____	50	25	155	5	2
473	Rye wafers, whole-grain, 1 ⅞ by 3 ½ inches.	2 wafers_____	13	6	45	2	Trace
474	Spaghetti, cooked, tender stage, enriched.	1 cup_____	140	72	155	5	1
	Spaghetti with meat balls, and tomato sauce:						
475	Home recipe_____ 1 cup_____		248	70	330	19	12
476	Canned_____ 1 cup_____		250	78	260	12	10
	Spaghetti in tomato sauce with cheese:						
477	Home recipe_____ 1 cup_____		250	77	260	9	9
478	Canned_____ 1 cup_____		250	80	190	6	2
479	Waffles, with enriched flour, 7-in. diam.	1 waffle_____	75	41	210	7	7
480	Waffles, made from mix, enriched, egg and milk added, 7-in. diam.	1 waffle_____	75	42	205	7	8
481	Wheat, puffed, added nutrients.	1 cup_____	15	3	55	2	Trace
482	Wheat, shredded, plain___ 1 biscuit_____		25	7	90	2	1
483	Wheat flakes, added nutrients.	1 cup_____	30	4	105	3	Trace
	Wheat flours:						
484	Whole-wheat, from hard wheats, stirred.	1 cup_____	120	12	400	16	2
	All-purpose or family flour, enriched:						
485	Sifted_____ 1 cup_____		115	12	420	12	1
486	Unsifted_____ 1 cup_____		125	12	455	13	1
487	Self-rising, enriched____ 1 cup_____		125	12	440	12	1
488	Cake or pastry flour, sifted.	1 cup_____	96	12	350	7	1

THE EDIBLE PART OF FOODS—Continued

there is reason tò believe that a measurable amount of the nutrient may be present]

Fatty acids			Carbohydrate	Calcium	Iron	Vitamin A value	Thiamin	Riboflavin	Niacin	Ascorbic acid
Saturated (total)	Unsaturated									
	Oleic	Linoleic								
Grams	*Grams*	*Grams*	*Grams*	*Milligrams*	*Milligrams*	*International units*	*Milligrams*	*Milligrams*	*Milligrams*	*Milligrams*
Trace	1	Trace	30	24	1.2	Trace	.13	.12	1.4	Trace
------	------	------	10	7	.5	0	.04	.03	.2	0
------	------	------	32	11	[19]1.3	0	[19].20	[19].11	[19]1.5	0
4	6	1	39	124	3.7	1,590	0.25	0.30	4.0	22
2	3	4	28	53	3.3	1,000	.15	.18	2.3	5
2	5	1	37	80	2.3	1,080	.25	.18	2.3	13
1	1	1	38	40	2.8	930	.35	.28	4.5	10
2	4	1	28	85	1.3	250	.13	.19	1.0	Trace
3	3	1	27	179	1.0	170	.11	.17	.7	Trace
------	------	------	12	4	.6	0	.08	.03	1.2	0
------	------	------	20	11	.9	0	.06	.03	1.1	0
------	------	------	24	12	1.3	0	.19	.04	1.5	0
Trace	1	1	85	49	4.0	0	.66	.14	5.2	0
------	------	------	88	18	[19]3.3	0	[19].51	[19].30	[19]4.0	0
------	------	------	95	20	[19]3.6	0	[19].55	[19].33	[19]4.4	0
------	------	------	93	331	[19]3.6	0	[19].55	[19].33	[19]4.4	0
------	------	------	76	16	.5	0	.03	.03	.7	0

TABLE 1.—NUTRITIVE VALUES OF

[Dashes in the columns for nutrients show that no suitable value could be found although

	Food, approximate measure, and weight (in grams)	Water	Food energy	Protein	Fat
	FATS, OILS				
		Grams	*Per-cent*	*Calo-ries*	*Grams*	*Grams*
	Butter:					
	Regular, 4 sticks per pound:					
489	Stick_____ ½ cup_____	113	16	810	1	92
490	Tablespoon (approx. 1 tbsp._____ ⅛ stick).	14	16	100	Trace	12
491	Pat (1-in. sq. ⅓-in. 1 pat_____ high; 90 per lb.).	5	16	35	Trace	4
	Whipped, 6 sticks or 2, 8-oz. containers per pound:					
492	Stick_____ ½ cup_____	76	16	540	1	61
493	Tablespoon (approx. 1 tbsp._____ ⅛ stick).	9	16	65	Trace	8
494	Pat (1¼-in. sq. ⅓-in. 1 pat_____ high; 120 per lb.).	4	16	25	Trace	3
	Fats, cooking:					
495	Lard_____ 1 cup_____	205	0	1,850	0	205
496	1 tbsp._____	13	0	115	0	13
497	Vegetable fats_____ 1 cup_____	200	0	1,770	0	200
498	1 tbsp._____	13	0	110	0	13
	Margarine:					
	Regular, 4 sticks per pound:					
499	Stick_____ ½ cup_____	113	16	815	1	92
500	Tablespoon (approx. 1 tbsp._____ ⅛ stick).	14	16	100	Trace	12
501	Pat (1-in. sq. ⅓-in. 1 pat_____ high; 90 per lb.).	5	16	35	Trace	4
	Whipped, 6 sticks per pound:					
502	Stick_____ ½ cup_____	76	16	545	1	61
	Soft, 2 8-oz. tubs per pound:					
503	Tub_____ 1 tub_____	227	16	1,635	1	184
504	Tablespoon_____ 1 tbsp._____	14	16	100	Trace	11

THE EDIBLE PART OF FOODS—Continued

there is reason to believe that a measurable amount of the nutrient may be present]

Fatty acids			Carbo-hy-drate	Cal-cium	Iron	Vita-min A value	Thia-min	Ribo-flavin	Niacin	Ascor-bic acid
Satu-rated (total)	Unsaturated									
	Oleic	Lin-oleic								
Grams	*Grams*	*Grams*	*Grams*	*Milli-grams*	*Milli-grams*	*Inter-national units*	*Milli-grams*	*Milli-grams*	*Milli-grams*	*Milli-grams*
51	30	3	1	23	0	[21]3,750	------	------	------	0
6	4	Trace	Trace	3	0	[21]470	------	------	------	0
2	1	Trace	Trace	1	0	[21]170	------	------	------	0
34	20	2	Trace	15	0	[21]2,500	------	------	------	0
4	3	Trace	Trace	2	0	[21]310	------	------	------	0
2	1	Trace	Trace	1	0	[21]130	------	------	------	0
78	94	20	0	0	0	0	0	0	0	0
5	6	1	0	0	0	0	0	0	0	0
50	100	44	0	0	0	------	0	0	0	0
3	6	3	0	0	0	------	0	0	0	0
17	46	25	1	23	0	[22]3,750	------	------	------	0
2	6	3	Trace	3	0	[22]470	------	------	------	0
1	2	1	Trace	1	0	[22]170	------	------	------	0
11	31	17	Trace	15	0	[22]2,500	------	------	------	0
34	68	68	1	45	0	[22]7,500	------	------	------	0
2	4	4	Trace	3	0	[22]470	------	------	------	0

TABLE 1.—NUTRITIVE VALUES OF

[Dashes in the columns for nutrients show that no suitable value could be found although

	Food, approximate measure, and weight (in grams)		Water	Food energy	Pro-tein	Fat
		Grams	Per-cent	Calo-ries	Grams	Grams
	FATS, OILS—Continued					
	Oils, salad or cooking:					
505	Corn_____ 1 cup_____	220	0	1,945	0	220
506	1 tbsp._____	14	0	125	0	14
507	Cottonseed_____ 1 cup_____	220	0	1,945	0	220
508	1 tbsp._____	14	0	125	0	14
509	Olive_____ 1 cup_____	220	0	1,945	0	220
510	1 tbsp._____	14	0	125	0	14
511	Peanut_____ 1 cup_____	220	0	1,945	0	220
512	1 tbsp._____	14	0	125	0	14
513	Safflower_____ 1 cup_____	220	0	1,945	0	220
514	1 tbsp._____	14	0	125	0	14
515	Soybean_____ 1 cup_____	220	0	1,945	0	220
516	1 tbsp._____	14	0	125	0	14
	Salad dressings:					
517	Blue cheese_____ 1 tbsp._____	15	32	75	1	8
	Commercial, mayonnaise type:					
518	Regular_____ 1 tbsp._____	15	41	65	Trace	6
519	Special dietary, low- 1 tbsp._____ calorie.	16	81	20	Trace	2
	French:					
520	Regular_____ 1 tbsp._____	16	39	65	Trace	6
521	Special dietary, low- 1 tbsp._____ fat with artificial sweeteners.	15	95	Trace	Trace	Trace
522	Home cooked, boiled_____ 1 tbsp.____	16	68	25	1	2
523	Mayonnaise_____ 1 tbsp.____	14	15	100	Trace	11
524	Thousand island_____ 1 tbsp.____	16	32	80	Trace	8
	SUGARS, SWEETS					
	Cake icings:					
525	Chocolate made with 1 cup_____	275	14	1,035	9	38

THE EDIBLE PART OF FOODS—Continued

there is reason to believe that a measurable amount of the nutrient may be present]

Fatty acids			Carbo-hy-drate	Cal-cium	Iron	Vita-min A value	Thia-min	Ribo-flavin	Niacin	Ascor-bic acid
Satu-rated (total)	Unsaturated									
	Oleic	Lin-oleic								
Grams	*Grams*	*Grams*	*Grams*	*Milli-grams*	*Milli-grams*	*Inter-national units*	*Milli-grams*	*Milli-grams*	*Milli-grams*	*Milli-grams*
22	62	117	0	0	0	-------	0	0	0	0
1	4	7	0	0	0	-------	0	0	0	0
55	46	110	0	0	0	-------	0	0	0	0
4	3	7	0	0	0	-------	0	0	0	0
24	167	15	0	0	0	-------	0	0	0	0
2	11	1	0	0	0	-------	0	0	0	0
40	103	64	0	0	0	-------	0	0	0	0
3	7	4	0	0	0	-------	0	0	0	0
18	37	165	0	0	0	-------	0	0	0	0
1	2	10	0	0	0	-------	0	0	0	0
33	44	114	0	0	0	-------	0	0	0	0
2	3	7	0	0	0	-------	0	0	0	0
2	2	4	1	12	Trace	30	Trace	0.02	Trace	Trace
1	1	3	2	2	Trace	30	Trace	Trace	Trace	------
Trace	Trace	1	1	3	Trace	40	Trace	Trace	Trace	------
1	1	3	3	2	.1	-------	-------	-------	-------	------
------	------	------	Trace	2	.1	-------	-------	-------	-------	------
1	1	Trace	2	14	.1	80	.01	.03	Trace	Trace
2	2	6	Trace	3	.1	40	Trace	.01	Trace	------
1	2	4	3	2	.1	50	Trace	Trace	Trace	Trace
21	14	1	185	165	3.3	580	.06	.28	.6	1

TABLE 1.—NUTRITIVE VALUES OF

[Dashes in the columns for nutrients show that no suitable value could be found although

	Food, approximate measure, and weight (in grams)			Water	Food energy	Pro-tein	Fat
			Grams	Per-cent	Calo-ries	Grams	Grams
	SUGARS, SWEETS—Continued						
	milk and table fat.						
526	Coconut (with boiled icing).	1 cup_____	166	15	605	3	13
527	Creamy fudge from mix with water only.	1 cup_____	245	15	830	7	16
528	White, boiled_____	1 cup_____	94	18	300	1	0
	Candy:						
529	Caramels, plain or chocolate.	1 oz._____	28	8	115	1	3
530	Chocolate, milk, plain__	1 oz._____	28	1	145	2	9
531	Chocolate-coated peanuts.	1 oz._____	28	1	160	5	12
532	Fondant; mints, un-coated; candy corn.	1 oz._____	28	8	105	Trace	1
533	Fudge, plain_____	1 oz._____	28	8	115	1	4
534	Gum drops_____	1 oz._____	28	12	100	Trace	Trace
535	Hard_____	1 oz._____	28	1	110	0	Trace
536	Marshmallows_____	1 oz._____	28	17	90	1	Trace
	Chocolate-flavored sirup or topping:						
537	Thin type_____	1 fl. oz._____	38	32	90	1	1
538	Fudge type_____	1 fl. oz._____	38	25	125	2	5
	Chocolate-flavored beverage powder (approx. 4 heaping teaspoons per oz.):						
539	With nonfat dry milk__	1 oz._____	28	2	100	5	1
540	Without nonfat dry milk.	1 oz._____	28	1	100	1	1
541	Honey, strained or extracted.	1 tbsp._____	21	17	65	Trace	0
542	Jams and preserves_____	1 tbsp._____	20	29	55	Trace	Trace
543	Jellies_____	1 tbsp._____	18	29	50	Trace	Trace

THE EDIBLE PART OF FOODS—Continued

there is reason to believe that a measurable amount of the nutrient may be present]

Fatty acids			Carbo-hy-drate	Cal-cium	Iron	Vita-min A value	Thia-min	Ribo-flavin	Niacin	Ascor-bic acid
Satu-rated (total)	Unsaturated									
	Oleic	Lin-oleic								
Grams	*Grams*	*Grams*	*Grams*	*Milli-grams*	*Milli-grams*	*Inter-national units*	*Milli-grams*	*Milli-grams*	*Milli-grams*	*Milli-grams*
11	1	Trace	124	10	.8	0	.02	.07	.3	0
5	8	3	183	96	2.7	Trace	.05	.20	.7	Trace
------	------	------	76	2	Trace	0	Trace	.03	Trace	0
2	1	Trace	22	42	.4	Trace	.01	.05	.1	Trace
5	3	Trace	16	65	.3	80	.02	.10	.1	Trace
3	6	2	11	33	.4	Trace	.10	.05	2.1	Trace
------	------	------	25	4	.3	0	Trace	Trace	Trace	0
2	1	Trace	21	22	.3	Trace	.01	.03	.1	Trace
------	------	------	25	2	.1	0	0	Trace	Trace	0
------	------	------	28	6	.5	0	0	0	0	0
------	------	------	23	5	.5	0	0	Trace	Trace	0
Trace	Trace	Trace	24	6	.6	Trace	.01	.03	.2	0
3	2	Trace	20	48	.5	60	.02	.08	.2	Trace
Trace	Trace	Trace	20	167	.5	10	.04	.21	.2	1
Trace	Trace	Trace	25	9	.6	------	.01	.03	.1	0
------	------	------	17	1	.1	0	Trace	.01	.1	Trace
------	------	------	14	4	.2	Trace	Trace	.01	Trace	Trace
------	------	------	13	4	.3	Trace	Trace	.01	Trace	1

TABLE 1.—NUTRITIVE VALUES OF

[Dashes in the columns for nutrients show that no suitable value could be found although

	Food, approximate measure, and weight (in grams)			Water	Food energy	Pro-tein	Fat
			Grams	*Per-cent*	*Calo-ries*	*Grams*	*Grams*
	SUGARS, SWEETS—Continued						
	Molasses, cane:						
544	Light (first extraction)	1 tbsp.	20	24	50	------	------
545	Blackstrap (third extraction).	1 tbsp.	20	24	45	------	------
	Sirups:						
546	Sorghum	1 tbsp.	21	23	55	------	------
547	Table blends, chiefly corn, light and dark.	1 tbsp.	21	24	60	0	0
	Sugars:						
548	Brown, firm packed	1 cup	220	2	820	0	0
	White:						
549	Granulated	1 cup	200	Trace	770	0	0
550		1 tbsp.	11	Trace	40	0	0
551	Powdered, stirred before measuring.	1 cup	120	Trace	460	0	0
	MISCELLANEOUS ITEMS						
552	Barbecue sauce	1 cup	250	81	230	4	17
	Beverages, alcoholic:						
553	Beer	12 fl. oz.	360	92	150	1	0
	Gin, rum, vodka, whiskey:						
554	80-proof	1½ fl. oz. jigger.	42	67	100	------	------
555	86-proof	1½ fl. oz. jigger.	42	64	105	------	------
556	90-proof	1½ fl. oz. jigger.	42	62	110	------	------
557	94-proof	1½ fl. oz. jigger.	42	60	115	------	------
558	100-proof	1½ fl. oz. jigger.	42	58	125	------	------

THE EDIBLE PART OF FOODS—Continued

there is reason to believe that a measurable amount of the nutrient may be present]

Fatty acids			Carbo-hydrate	Cal-cium	Iron	Vita-min A value	Thia-min	Ribo-flavin	Niacin	Ascorbic acid
Satu-rated (total)	Unsaturated									
	Oleic	Lin-oleic								
Grams	*Grams*	*Grams*	*Grams*	*Milligrams*	*Milligrams*	*International units*	*Milligrams*	*Milligrams*	*Milligrams*	*Milligrams*
------	------	------	13	33	.9	------	.01	.01	Trace	------
------	------	------	11	137	3.2	------	.02	.04	.4	------
------	------	------	14	35	2.6	------	------	.02	Trace	------
------	------	------	15	9	.8	0	0	0	0	0
------	------	------	212	187	7.5	0	.02	.07	.4	0
------	------	------	199	0	.2	0	0	0	0	0
------	------	------	11	0	Trace	0	0	0	0	0
------	------	------	119	0	.1	0	0	0	0	0
2	5	9	20	53	2.0	900	.03	.03	.8	13
------	------	------	14	18	Trace	------	.01	.11	2.2	------
------	------	------	Trace	------	------	------	------	------	------	------
------	------	------	Trace	------	------	------	------	------	------	------
------	------	------	Trace	------	------	------	------	------	------	------
------	------	------	Trace	------	------	------	------	------	------	------
------	------	------	Trace	------	------	------	------	------	------	------

TABLE 1.—NUTRITIVE VALUES OF

[Dashes in the columns for nutrients show that no suitable value could be found although

	Food, approximate measure, and weight (in grams)			Water	Food energy	Pro-tein	Fat
			Grams	*Per-cent*	*Calo-ries*	*Grams*	*Grams*
	MISCELLANEOUS ITEMS—Continued						
	Wines:						
559	Dessert_____	3½ fl. oz. glass.	103	77	140	Trace	0
560	Table_____	3½ fl. oz. glass.	102	86	85	Trace	0
	Beverages, carbonated, sweetened, nonalcoholic:						
561	Carbonated water_____	12 fl. oz._____	366	92	115	0	0
562	Cola type_____	12 fl. oz._____	369	90	145	0	0
563	Fruit-flavored sodas and Tom Collins mixes.	12 fl. oz._____	372	88	170	0	0
564	Ginger ale_____	12 fl. oz._____	366	92	115	0	0
565	Root beer_____	12 fl. oz._____	370	90	150	0	0
566	Bouillon cubes, approx. ½ in.	1 cube_____	4	4	5	1	Trace
	Chocolate:						
567	Bitter or baking_____	1 oz._____	28	2	145	3	15
568	Semi-sweet, small pieces.	1 cup_____	170	1	860	7	61
	Gelatin:						
569	Plain, dry powder in envelope.	1 envelope___	7	13	25	6	Trace
570	Dessert powder, 3-oz. package.	1 pkg._____	85	2	315	8	0
571	Gelatin dessert, prepared with water.	1 cup_____	240	84	140	4	0
	Olives, pickled:						
572	Green_____	4 medium or 3 extra large or 2 giant.	16	78	15	Trace	2
573	Ripe: Mission_____	3 small or 2 large.	10	73	15	Trace	

THE EDIBLE PART OF FOODS—Continued

there is reason to believe that a measurable amount of the nutrient may be present]

Fatty acids			Carbo-hy-drate	Cal-cium	Iron	Vita-min A value	Thia-min	Ribo-flavin	Niacin	Ascor-bic acid
Satu-rated (total)	Unsaturated									
	Oleic	Lin-oleic								
Grams	*Grams*	*Grams*	*Grams*	*Milli-grams*	*Milli-grams*	*Inter-national units*	*Milli-grams*	*Milli-grams*	*Milli-grams*	*Milli-grams*
------	------	------	8	8	------	------	.01	.02	.2	------
------	------	------	4	9	.4	------	Trace	.01	.1	------
------	------	------	29	------	------	0	0	0	0	0
------	------	------	37	------	------	0	0	0	0	0
------	------	------	45	------	------	0	0	0	0	0
------	------	------	29	------	------	0	0	0	0	0
------	------	------	39	------	------	0	0	0	0	0
------	------	------	Trace	------	------	------	------	------	------	------
8	6	Trace	8	22	1.9	20	.01	.07	.4	0
34	22	1	97	51	4.4	30	.02	.14	.9	0
------	------	------	0	------	------	------	------	------	------	------
------	------	------	75	------	------	------	------	------	------	------
------	------	------	34	------	------	------	------	------	------	------
Trace	2	Trace	Trace	8	.2	40	------	------	------	------
Trace	2	Trace	Trace	9	.1	10	Trace	Trace	------	------

TABLE 1.—NUTRITIVE VALUES OF

[Dashes in the columns for nutrients show that no suitable value could be found although

	Food, approximate measure, and weight (in grams)			Water	Food energy	Pro-tein	Fat
			Grams	Per-cent	Calo-ries	Grams	Grams
	MISCELLANEOUS ITEMS—Continued						
	Pickles, cucumber:						
574	Dill, medium, whole, 3¾ in. long, 1¼ in. diam.	1 pickle_____	65	93	10	1	Trace
575	Fresh, sliced, 1½ in. diam., ¼ in. thick.	2 slices_____	15	79	10	Trace	Trace
576	Sweet, gherkin, small, whole, approx. 2½ in. long, ¾ in. diam.	1 pickle_____	15	61	20	Trace	Trace
577	Relish, finely chopped, sweet.	1 tbsp._____	15	63	20	Trace	Trace
	Popcorn. See Grain Products.						
578	Popsicle, 3 fl. oz. size____	1 popsicle____	95	80	70	0	0
	Pudding, home recipe with starch base:						
579	Chocolate_____	1 cup_____	260	66	385	8	12
580	Vanilla (blanc mange)__	1 cup_____	255	76	285	9	10
581	Pudding mix, dry form, 4-oz. package.	1 pkg._____	113	2	410	3	2
582	Sherbet_____	1 cup_____	193	67	260	2	2
	Soups:						
	Canned, condensed, ready-to-serve:						
	Prepared with an equal volume of milk:						
583	Cream of chicken__	1 cup_____	245	85	180	7	10
584	Cream of mush-room.	1 cup_____	245	83	215	7	14
585	Tomato_____	1 cup_____	250	84	175	7	7
	Prepared with an equal volume of water:						
586	Bean with pork___	1 cup_____	250	84	170	8	6
587	Beef broth, bouil-lon consomme.	1 cup_____	240	96	30	5	0
588	Beef noodle_____	1 cup_____	240	93	70	4	3

THE EDIBLE PART OF FOODS—Continued

there is reason to believe that a measurable amount of the nutrient may be present]

Fatty acids			Carbo-hy-drate	Cal-cium	Iron	Vita-min A value	Thia-min	Ribo-flavin	Niacin	Ascor-bic acid
Satu-rated (total)	Unsaturated									
	Oleic	Lin-oleic								
Grams	*Grams*	*Grams*	*Grams*	*Milli-grams*	*Milli-grams*	*Inter-national units*	*Milli-grams*	*Milli-grams*	*Milli-grams*	*Milli-grams*
------	------	------	1	17	.7	70	Trace	.01	Trace	4
------	------	------	3	5	.3	20	Trace	Trace	Trace	1
------	------	------	6	2	.2	10	Trace	Trace	Trace	1
------	------	------	5	3	.1	------	------	------	------	------
0	0	0	18	0	Trace	0	0	0	0	0
7	4	Trace	67	250	1.3	390	.05	.36	.3	1
5	3	Trace	41	298	Trace	410	.08	.41	.3	2
1	1	Trace	103	23	1.8	Trace	.02	.08	.5	0
------	------	------	59	31	Trace	120	.02	.06	Trace	4
3	3	3	15	172	.5	610	.05	.27	.7	2
4	4	5	16	191	.5	250	.05	.34	.7	1
3	2	1	23	168	.8	1,200	.10	.25	1.3	15
1	2	2	22	63	2.3	650	.13	.08	1.0	3
			3	Trace	.5	Trace	Trace	.02	1.2	------
1	1	1	7	7	1.0	50	.05	.07	1.0	Trace

TABLE 1.—NUTRITIVE VALUES OF

[Dashes in the columns for nutrients show that no suitable value could be found although

Food, approximate measure, and weight (in grams)			Water	Food energy	Pro-tein	Fat
MISCELLANEOUS ITEMS—Continued						
		Grams	Per-cent	Calo-ries	Grams	Grams
589	Clam chowder, Manhattan type (with tomatoes, without milk).	1 cup_____ 245	92	80	2	3
590	Cream of chicken__	1 cup_____ 240	92	95	3	6
591	Cream of mush-room.	1 cup_____ 240	90	135	2	10
592	Minestrone_____	1 cup_____ 245	90	105	5	3
593	Split pea_____	1 cup_____ 245	85	145	9	3
594	Tomato_____	1 cup_____ 245	90	90	2	3
595	Vegetable beef____	1 cup_____ 245	92	80	5	2
596	Vegetarian_____	1 cup_____ 245	92	80	2	2
	Dehydrated, dry form:					
597	Chicken noodle (2-oz. package).	1 pkg._____ 57	6	220	8	6
598	Onion mix (1½-oz. package).	1 pkg._____ 43	3	150	6	5
599	Tomato vegetable with noodles (2½-oz. pkg.).	1 pkg._____ 71	4	245	6	6
	Frozen, condensed:					
	Clam chowder, New England type (with milk, without tomatoes):					
600	Prepared with equal volume of milk.	1 cup_____ 245	83	210	9	12
601	Prepared with equal volume of water.	1 cup_____ 240	89	130	4	8
	Cream of potato:					
602	Prepared with equal volume of milk.	1 cup_____ 245	83	185	8	10

THE EDIBLE PART OF FOODS—Continued

there is reason to believe that a measurable amount of the nutrient may be present]

Fatty acids			Carbo-hydrate	Cal-cium	Iron	Vita-min A value	Thia-min	Ribo-flavin	Niacin	Ascor-bic acid
Satu-rated (total)	Unsaturated									
	Oleic	Lin-oleic								
Grams	Grams	Grams	Grams	Milli-grams	Milli-grams	Inter-national units	Milli-grams	Milli-grams	Milli-grams	Milli-grams
------	------	------	12	34	1.0	880	.02	.02	1.0	------
1	2	3	8	24	.5	410	.02	.05	.5	Trace
1	3	5	10	41	.5	70	.02	.12	.7	Trace
------	------	------	14	37	1.0	2,350	.07	.05	1.0	------
1	2	Trace	21	29	1.5	440	0.25	0.15	1.5	1
Trace	1	1	16	15	.7	1,000	.05	.05	1.2	12
------	------	------	10	12	.7	2,700	.05	.05	1.0	------
------	------	------	13	20	1.0	2,940	.05	.05	1.0	------
2	3	1	33	34	1.4	190	.30	.15	2.4	3
1	2	1	23	42	.6	30	.05	.03	.3	6
2	3	1	45	33	1.4	1,700	.21	.13	1.8	18
------	------	------	16	240	1.0	250	.07	.29	.5	Trace
------	------	------	11	91	1.0	50	.05	.10	.5	------
5	3	Trace	18	208	1.0	590	.10	.27	.5	Trace

TABLE 1.—NUTRITIVE VALUES OF

[Dashes in the columns for nutrients show that no suitable value could be found although

	Food, approximate measure, and weight (in grams)			Water	Food energy	Pro- tein	Fat
	MISCELLANEOUS ITEMS—Continued		Grams	Per- cent	Calo- ries	Grams	Grams
603	Prepared with equal volume of water. Cream of shrimp:	1 cup	240	90	105	3	5
604	Prepared with equal volume of milk.	1 cup	245	82	245	9	16
605	Prepared with equal volume of water. Oyster stew:	1 cup	240	88	160	5	12
606	Prepared with equal volume of milk.	1 cup	240	83	200	10	12
607	Prepared with equal volume of water.	1 cup	240	90	120	6	8
608	Tapioca, dry, quick-cooking. Tapioca desserts:	1 cup	152	13	535	1	Trace
609	Apple	1 cup	250	70	295	1	Trace
610	Cream pudding	1 cup	165	72	220	8	8
611	Tartar sauce	1 tbsp.	14	34	75	Trace	8
612	Vinegar	1 tbsp.	15	94	Trace	Trace	0
613	White sauce, medium	1 cup	250	73	405	10	31
614	Yeast: Baker's, dry, active	1 pkg.	7	5	20	3	Trace
615	Brewer's, dry	1 tbsp.	8	5	25	3	Trace
	Yoghurt. See Milk, Cheese, Cream, Imitation Cream.						

THE EDIBLE PART OF FOODS—Continued

there is reason to believe that a measurable amount of the nutrient may be present]

Fatty acids			Carbo-hydrate	Cal-cium	Iron	Vita-min A value	Thia-min	Ribo-flavin	Niacin	Ascor-bic acid
Satu-rated (total)	Unsaturated									
	Oleic	Lin-oleic								
Grams	*Grams*	*Grams*	*Grams*	*Milli-grams*	*Milli-grams*	*Inter-national units*	*Milli-grams*	*Milli-grams*	*Milli-grams*	*Milli-grams*
3	2	Trace	12	58	1.0	410	.05	.05	.5	------
------	------	------	15	189	.5	290	.07	.27	.5	Trace
------	------	------	8	38	.5	120	.05	.05	.5	------
------	------	------	14	305	1.4	410	.12	.41	.5	Trace
------	------	------	8	158	1.4	240	.07	.19	.5	------
------	------	------	131	15	.6	0	0	0	0	0
------	------	------	74	8	.5	30	Trace	Trace	Trace	Trace
4	3	Trace	28	173	.7	480	.07	.30	.2	2
1	1	4	1	3	.1	30	Trace	Trace	Trace	Trace
------	------	------	1	1	.1	------	------	------	------	------
16	10	1	22	288	.5	1,150	.10	.43	.5	2
------	------	------	3	3	1.1	Trace	.16	.38	2.6	Trace
------	------	------	3	17	1.4	Trace	1.25	.34	3.0	Trace

TABLE 2.—RECOMMENDED DAILY

[Designed for the maintenance of good nutrition

Persons				Food energy	Protein
Age in years [3] *From up to*	*Weight in pounds*	*Height in inches*		*Calories*	*Grams*
Infants_____ 0–⅙_____	9_____	22_____		lb. x 54.5	lb. x 1.0
⅙–½_____	15_____	25_____		lb. x 50.0	lb. x .9
½–1_____	20_____	28_____		lb. x 45.5	lb. x .8
Children_____ 1–2_____	26_____	32_____		1,100	25
2–3_____	31_____	36_____		1,250	25
3–4_____	35_____	39_____		1,400	30
4–6_____	42_____	43_____		1,600	30
6–8_____	51_____	48_____		2,000	35
8–10_____	62_____	52_____		2,200	40
Boys_____ 10–12_____	77_____	55_____		2,500	45
12–14_____	95_____	59_____		2,700	50
14–18_____	130_____	67_____		3,000	60
Men_____ 18–22_____	147_____	69_____		2,800	60
22–35_____	154_____	69_____		2,800	65
35–55_____	154_____	68_____		2,600	65
55–75+____	154_____	67_____		2,400	65
Girls_____ 10–12_____	77_____	56_____		2,250	50
12–14_____	97_____	61_____		2,300	50
14–16_____	114_____	62_____		2,400	55
16–18_____	119_____	63_____		2,300	55
Women_____ 18–22_____	128_____	64_____		2,000	55
22–35_____	128_____	64_____		2,000	55
35–55_____	128_____	63_____		1,850	55
55–75+____	128_____	62_____		1,700	55
Pregnant_____				+200	65
Lactating_____				+1,000	75

DIETARY ALLOWANCES (ABRIDGED)[1]

of practically all healthy persons in the U.S.A.]

Calcium	Iron	Vitamin A	Thia-min	Ribo-flavin	Niacin equiva-lent [2]	Ascorbic acid
Grams	*Milli-grams*	*Interna-tional units*	*Milli-grams*	*Milli-grams*	*Milli-grams*	*Milli-grams*
0.4	6	1,500	0.2	0.4	5	35
0.5	10	1,500	0.4	0.5	7	35
0.6	15	1,500	0.5	0.6	8	35
0.7	15	2,000	0.6	0.6	8	40
0.8	15	2,000	0.6	0.7	8	40
0.8	10	2,500	0.7	0.8	9	40
0.8	10	2,500	0.8	0.9	11	40
0.9	10	3,500	1.0	1.1	13	40
1.0	10	3,500	1.1	1.2	15	40
1.2	10	4,500	1.3	1.3	17	40
1.4	18	5,000	1.4	1.4	18	45
1.4	18	5,000	1.5	1.5	20	55
0.8	10	5,000	1.4	1.6	18	60
0.8	10	5,000	1.4	1.7	18	60
0.8	10	5,000	1.3	1.7	17	60
0.8	10	5,000	1.2	1.7	14	60
1.2	18	4,500	1.1	1.3	15	40
1.3	18	5,000	1.2	1.4	15	45
1.3	18	5,000	1.2	1.4	16	50
1.3	18	5,000	1.2	1.5	15	50
0.8	18	5,000	1.0	1.5	13	55
0.8	18	5,000	1.0	1.5	13	55
0.8	18	5,000	1.0	1.5	13	55
0.8	10	5,000	1.0	1.5	13	55
+0.4	18	6,000	+0.1	1.8	15	60
+0.5	18	8,000	+0.5	2.0	20	60

REFERENCES—TABLE 1.

1. Value applies to unfortified product; value for fortified low-density product would be 1500 I.U. and the fortified high-density product would be 2290 I.U.

2. Contributed largely from beta-carotene used for coloring.

3. Outer layer of fat on the cut was removed to within approximately ½-inch of the lean. Deposits of fat within the cut were not removed.

4. If bones are discarded, value will be greatly reduced.

5. Measure and weight apply to entire vegetable or fruit including parts not usually eaten.

6. Based on yellow varieties; white varieties contain only a trace of cryptoxanthin and carotenes, the pigments in corn that have biological activity.

7. Year-round average. Samples marketed from November through May, average 20 milligrams per 200-gram tomato; from June through October, around 52 milligrams.

8. This is the amount from the fruit. Additional ascorbic acid may be added by the manufacturer. Refer to the label for this information.

9. Value for varieties with orange-colored flesh; value for varieties with green flesh would be about 540 I.U.

10. Value listed is based on products with label stating 30 milligrams per 6 fl. oz. serving.

11. For white-fleshed varieties value is about 20 I.U. per cup; for red-fleshed varieties, 1,080 I.U. per cup.

12. Present only if added by the manufacturer. Refer to the label for this information.

13. Based on yellow-fleshed varieties; for white-fleshed varieties value is about 50 I.U. per 114-gram peach and 80 I.U. per cup of sliced peaches.

14. This value includes ascorbic acid added by manufacturer.

15. Values for iron, thiamin, riboflavin, and niacin per pound of unenriched white bread would be as follows:

	Iron	Thiamin	Riboflavin	Niacin
	Milligrams	*Milligrams*	*Milligrams*	*Milligrams*
Soft crumb	3.2	.31	.39	5.0
Firm crumb	3.2	.32	.59	4.1

16. Unenriched cake flour used unless otherwise specified.

17. This value is based on product made from yellow varieties of corn; white varieties contain only a trace.

18. Based on product made with enriched flour. With unenriched flour, approximate values per doughnut are: Iron, 0.2 milligram; thiamin, 0.01 milligram; riboflavin, 0.03 milligram; niacin, 0.2 milligram.

19. Iron, thiamin, riboflavin, and niacin are based on the minimum levels of enrichment specified in standards of identity promulgated under the Federal Food, Drug, and Cosmetic Act.

20. Iron, thiamin, and niacin are based on the minimum levels of enrichment specified in standards of identity promulgated under the Federal Food, Drug, and Cosmetic Act. Riboflavin is based on unenriched rice. When the minimum level of enrichment for riboflavin specified in the standards of identity becomes effective the value will be 0.12 milligram per cup of parboiled rice and of white rice.

21. Year-round average.

22. Based on the average vitamin A content of fortified margarine. Federal specifications for fortified margarine require a minimum of 15,000 I.U. of Vitamin A per pound.

REFERENCES—TABLE 2.

1. Source: Adapted from Recommended Dietary Allowances, Seventh edition 1968, Publication 1694, 169 pages. Published by National Academy of Sciences—National Research Council, Washington, D.C. 20418. Also available in libraries. This publication includes discussion of allowances, eight additional nutrients, and adjustments needed for age, body size, and physical activity.

2. Niacin equivalents include dietary sources of the vitamin itself plus 1 milligram equivalent for each 60 milligrams of dietary tryptophan.

3. Entries for age range 22 to 35 years represent the reference man and woman at age 22. All other entries represent allowances for the midpoint of the specified age group.

NOTE.—The Recommended Daily Dietary Allowances should not be confused with Minimum Daily Requirements. The Recommended Dietary Allowances are amounts of nutrients recommended by the Food and Nutrition Board of National Research Council, and are considered adequate for maintenance of good nutrition in healthy persons in the United States. The allowances are revised from time to time in accordance with newer knowledge of nutritional needs.

The Minimum Daily Requirements are the amounts of selected nutrients that have been established by the Food and Drug Administration as standards for labeling purposes of foods and pharmaceutical preparations for special dietary uses. These are the amounts regarded as necessary in the diet for the prevention of deficiency diseases and generally are less than the Recommended Dietary Allowances. The Minimum Daily Requirements for the adult man are: Vitamin A, 4000 I.U.; thiamin, 1 milligram; riboflavin, 1.2 milligram; niacin, 10 milligrams; ascorbic acid, 30 milligrams; calcium, 750 milligrams; iron, 10 milligrams. For additional information on Minimum Daily Requirements see the Federal Register, vol. 6, No. 227 (Nov. 22, 1941), beginning on p. 5921, and amended as stated in the Federal Register (June 1, 1957), vol. 22, No. 106, p. 3841 (effective July 1, 1958).